Moving Your Way to a Great Big Smile!

A Beginner's Guide to Tai Chi for Little Ones

Ana Cybela

Illustrations by Widya Arumba

Printed in the United States of America
First Printing, 2020

Paperback: ISBN: 978-1-7355694-5-1
Hardcover: ISBN: 978-1-7355694-9-9

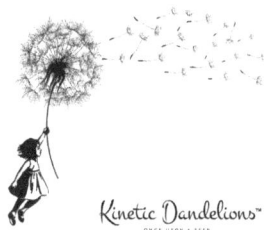

Kinetic Dandelions
ONCE UPON A SEED

For Sophie and Zoe

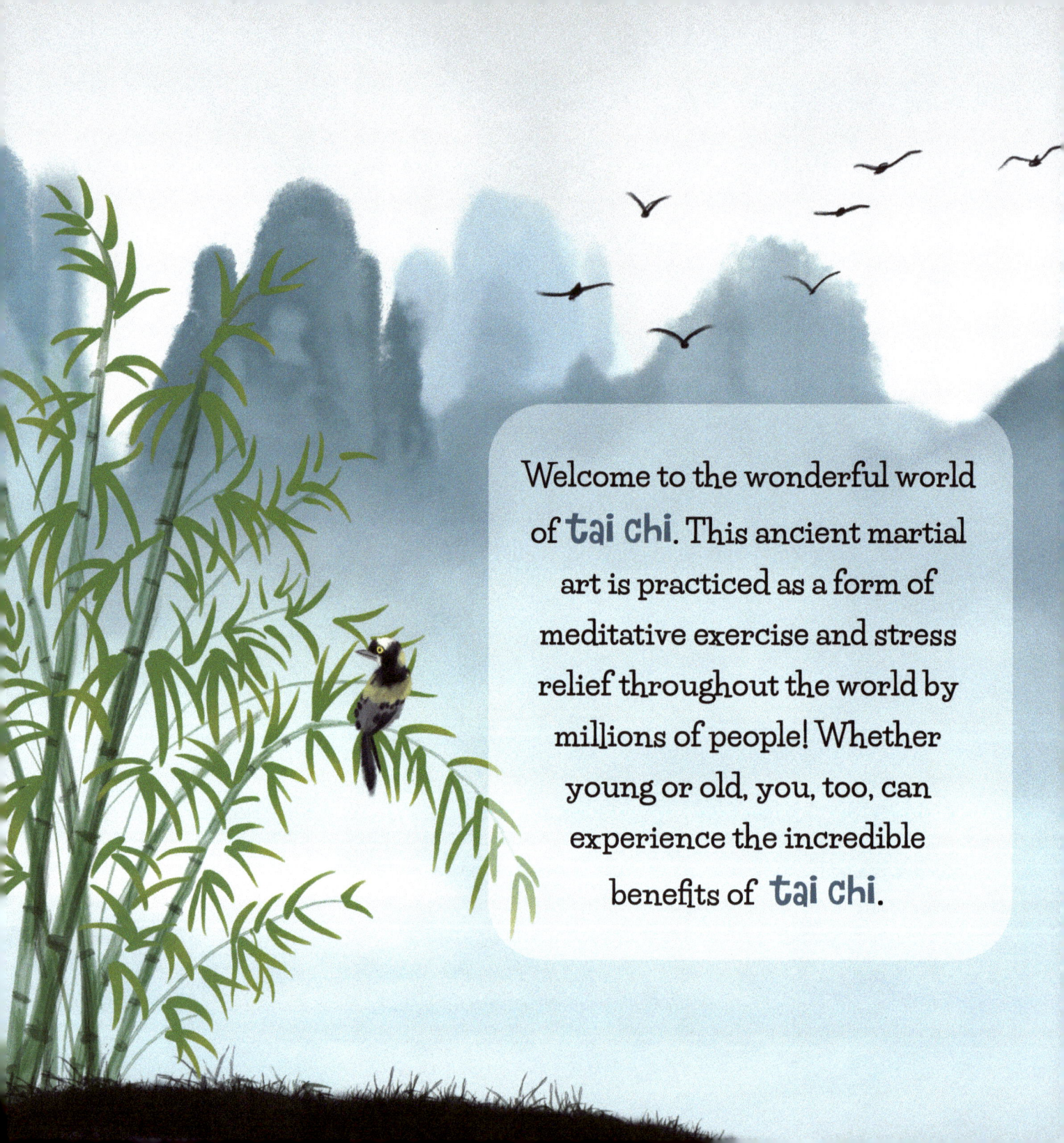

Welcome to the wonderful world of tai chi. This ancient martial art is practiced as a form of meditative exercise and stress relief throughout the world by millions of people! Whether young or old, you, too, can experience the incredible benefits of tai chi.

And now, *Moving Your Way to a Great Big Smile!* introduces fourteen tai chi moves to your little ones. Each move is based on either an animal or a natural object and is beautifully illustrated to entice even the youngest minds to give tai chi a try. If practiced daily, this mind-body exercise will help little ones feel their *qi* (pronounced *'chee'*), their life energy, flowing positively. So, dive into the practice of tai chi, discover the world of ancient Chinese wisdom and strength, and let the smiles begin!

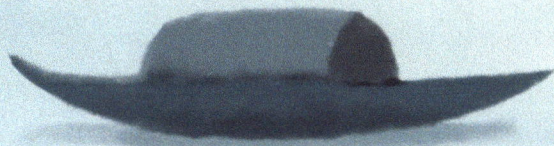

Stand tall and stretch far.
My feet root deeply into the ground.

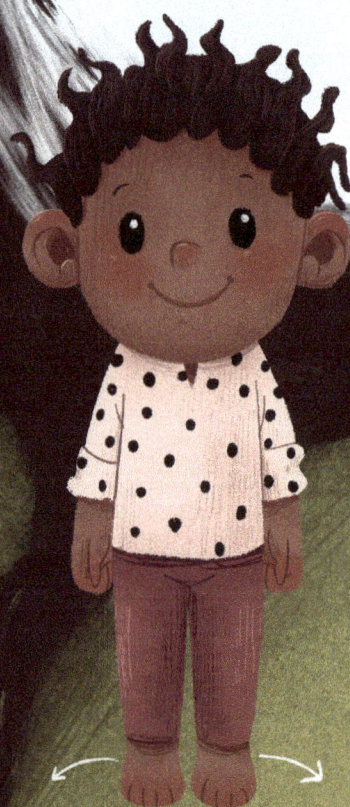

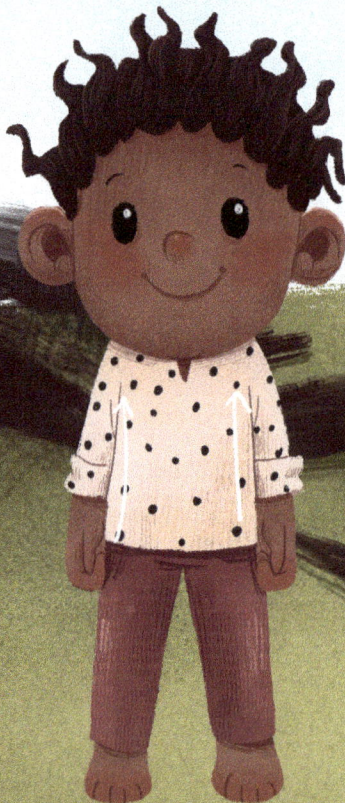

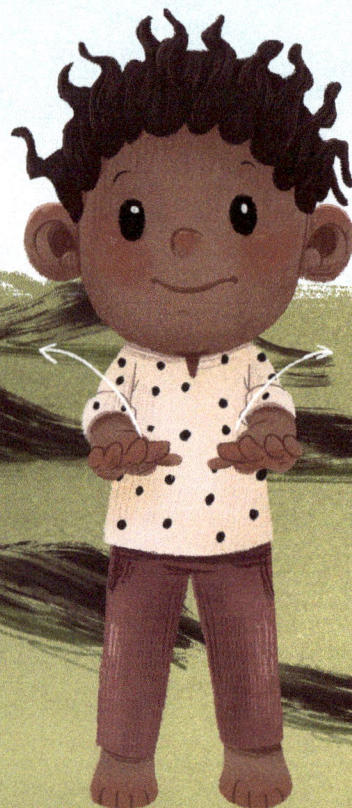

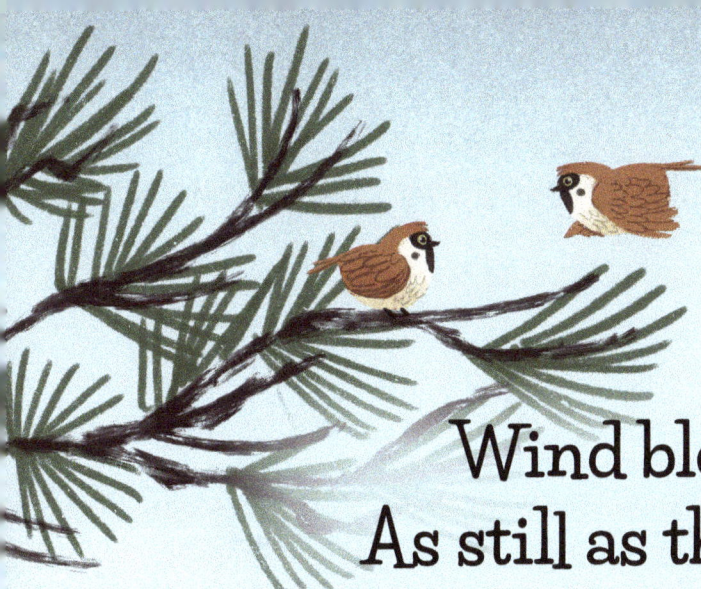

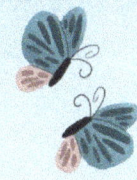

Wind blows. I am still.
As still as this big old **tree**.

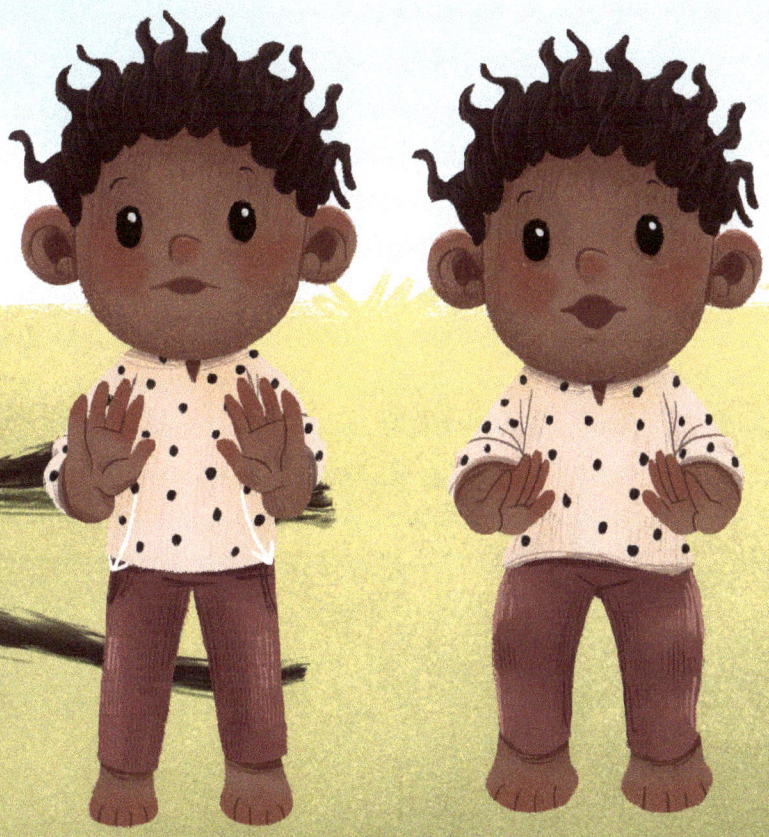

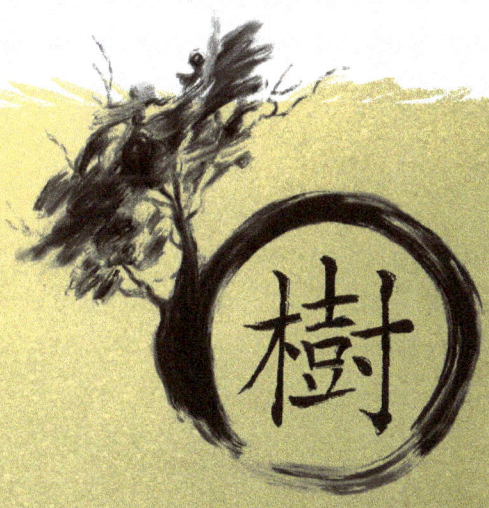

樹

Gallop away, here I come, moving like a **horse**, across the grass.

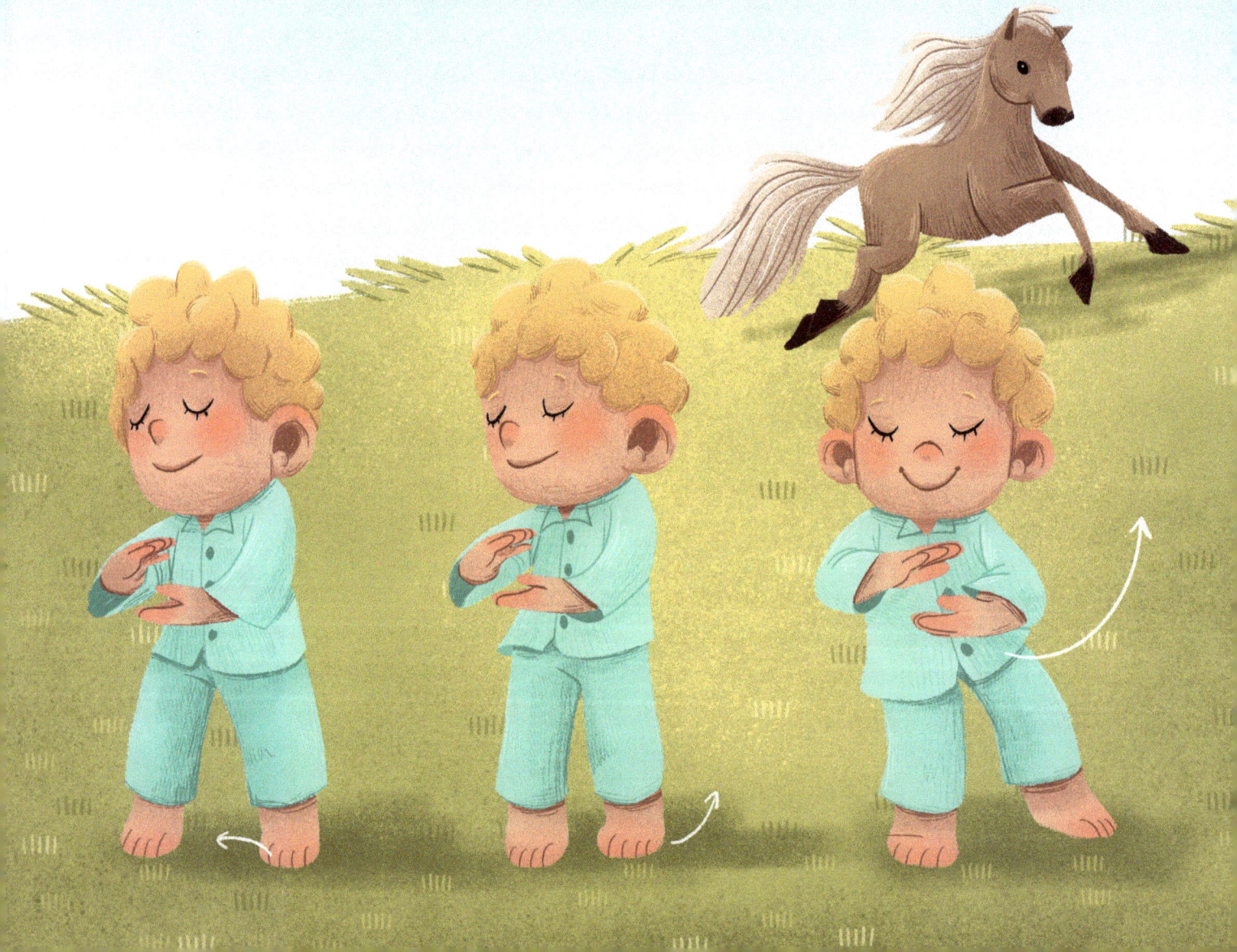

Feet forward, head high,
and away I sprint!

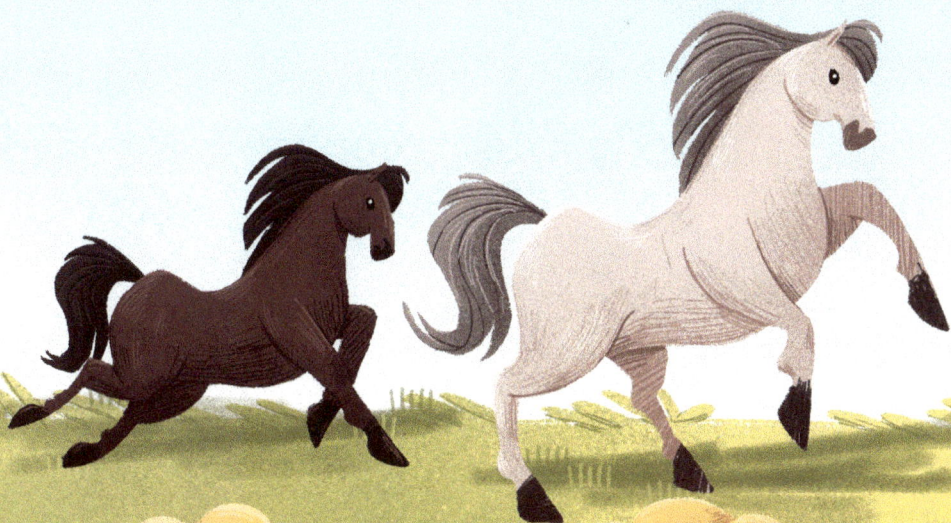

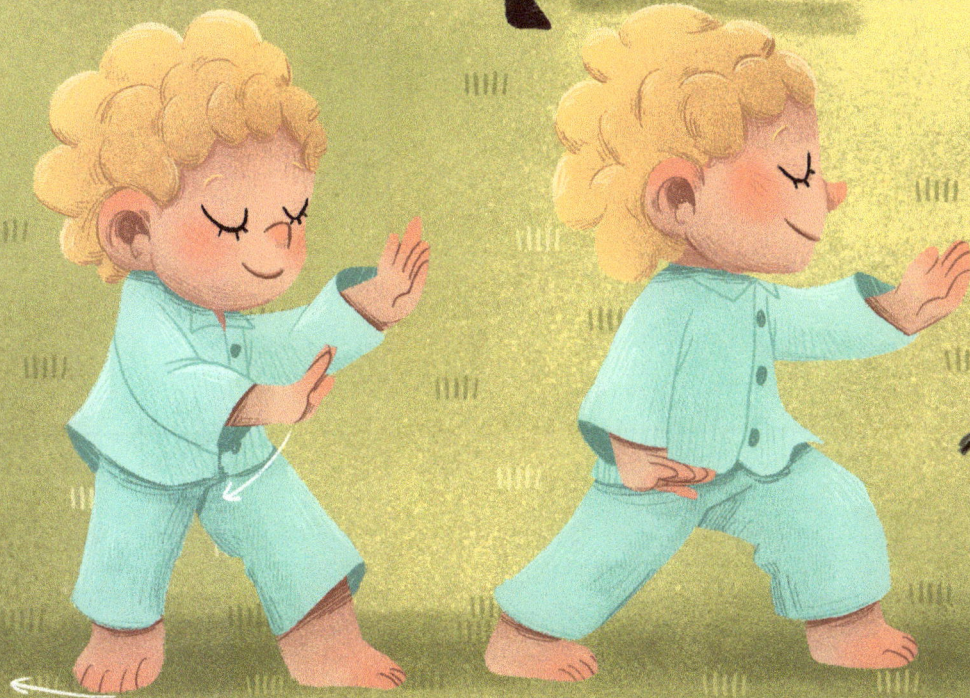

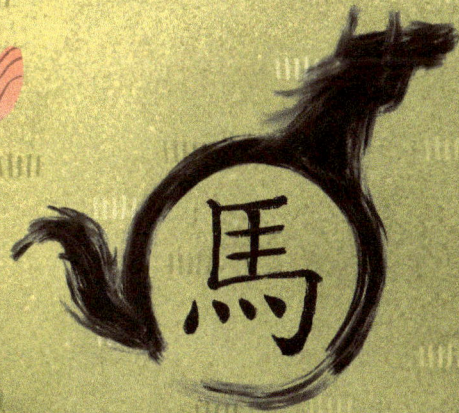

馬

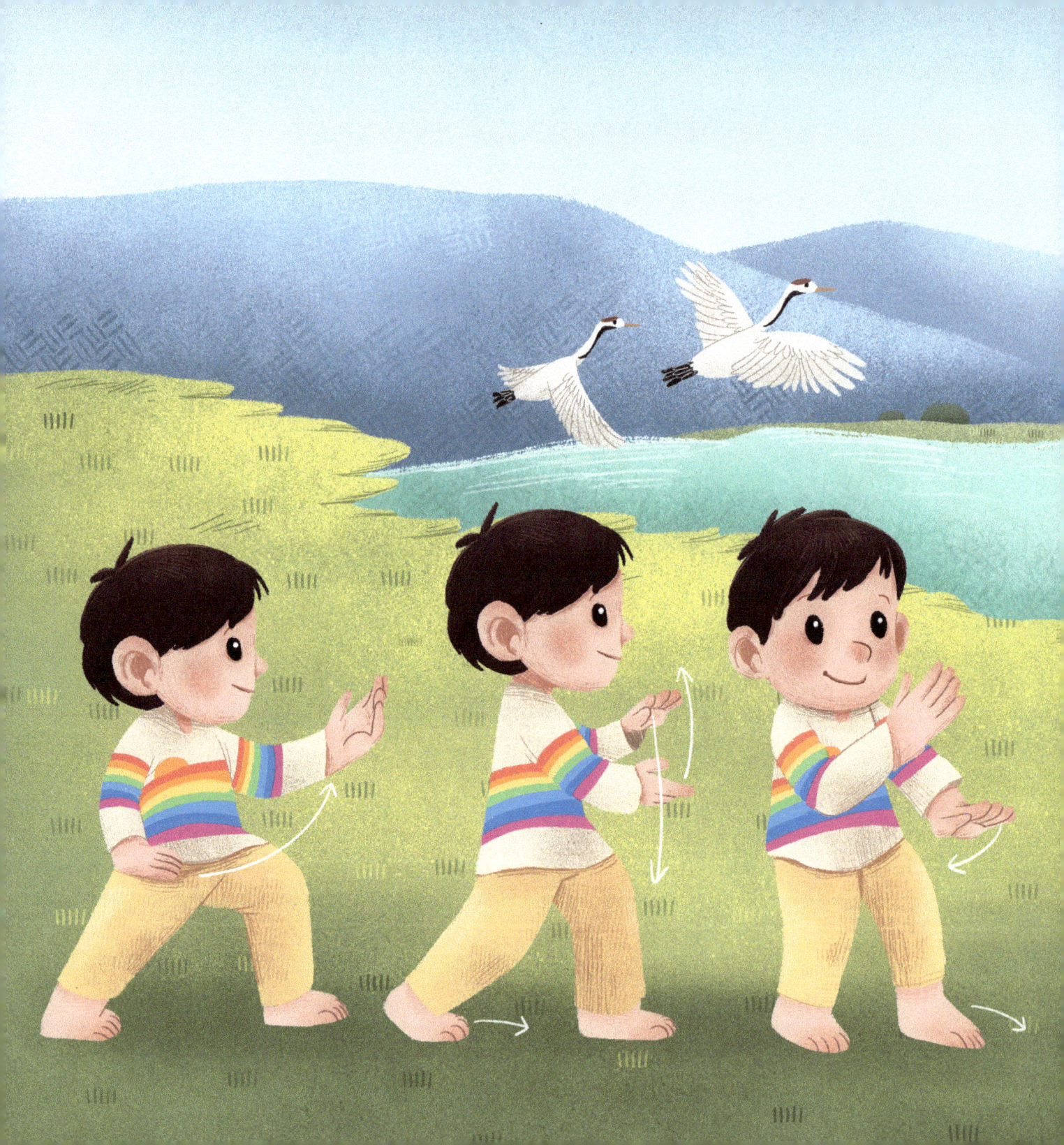

Crane, crane, flying away,
over the mountains, across the plains.

As I flap my wings,
I will soar and be free, too!

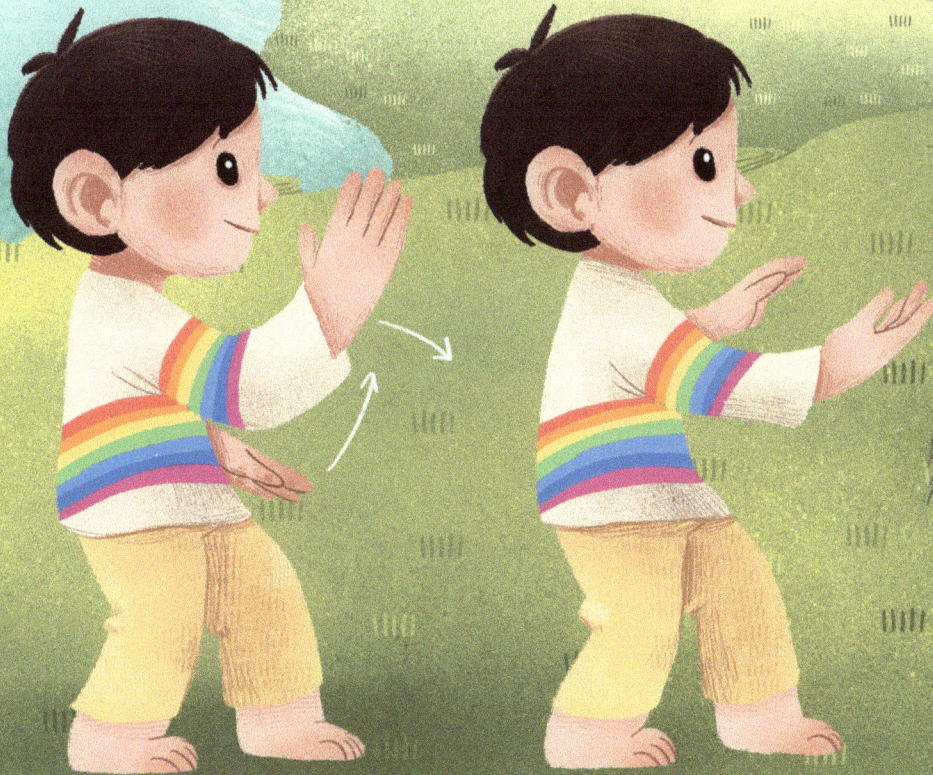

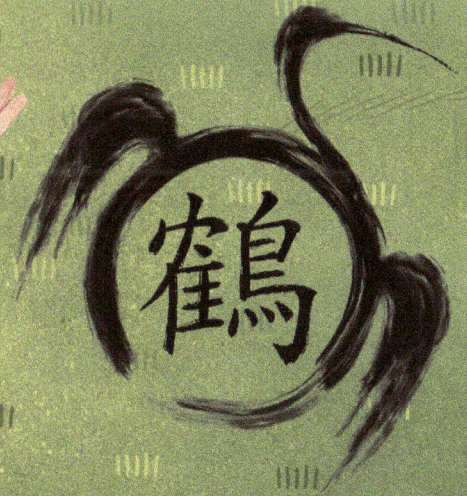

鶴

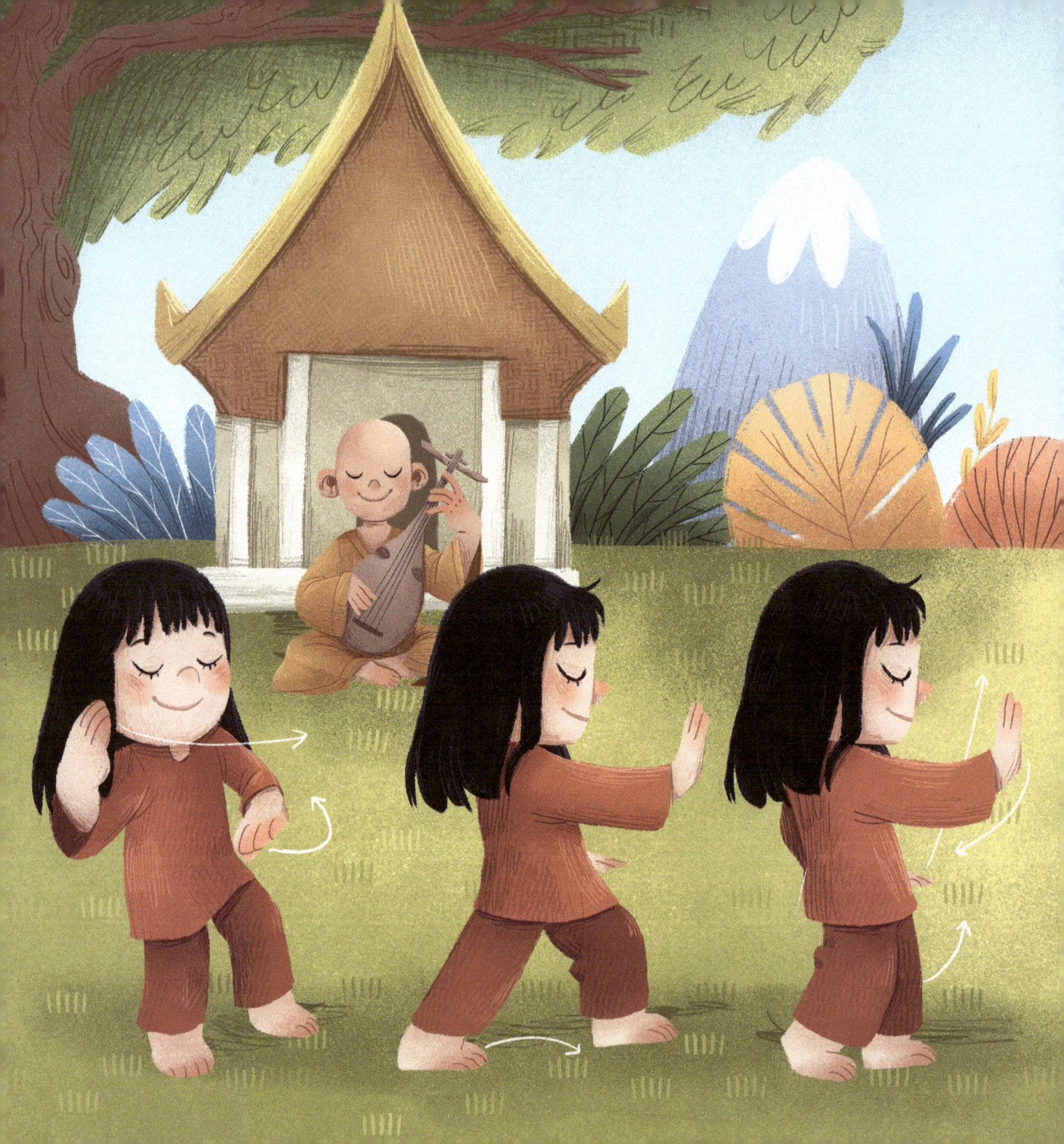

Sweet melody, Do, Re, Mi ...
slowly drifting nearby.

One, Two, Three ... I move my
arms and stretch my legs.
I can play the lute, too!

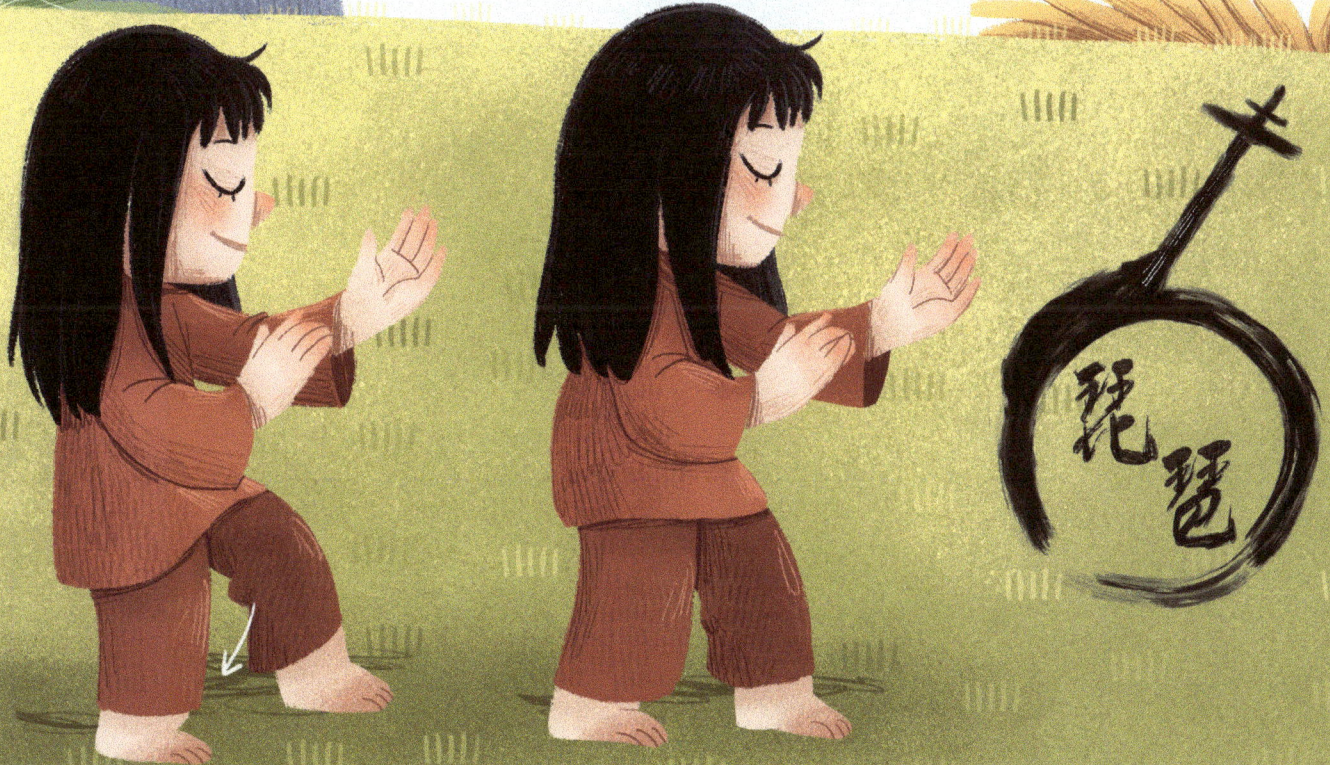

琵琶

Monkey see, monkey do!

Watch out, little monkey,
here I come for you!

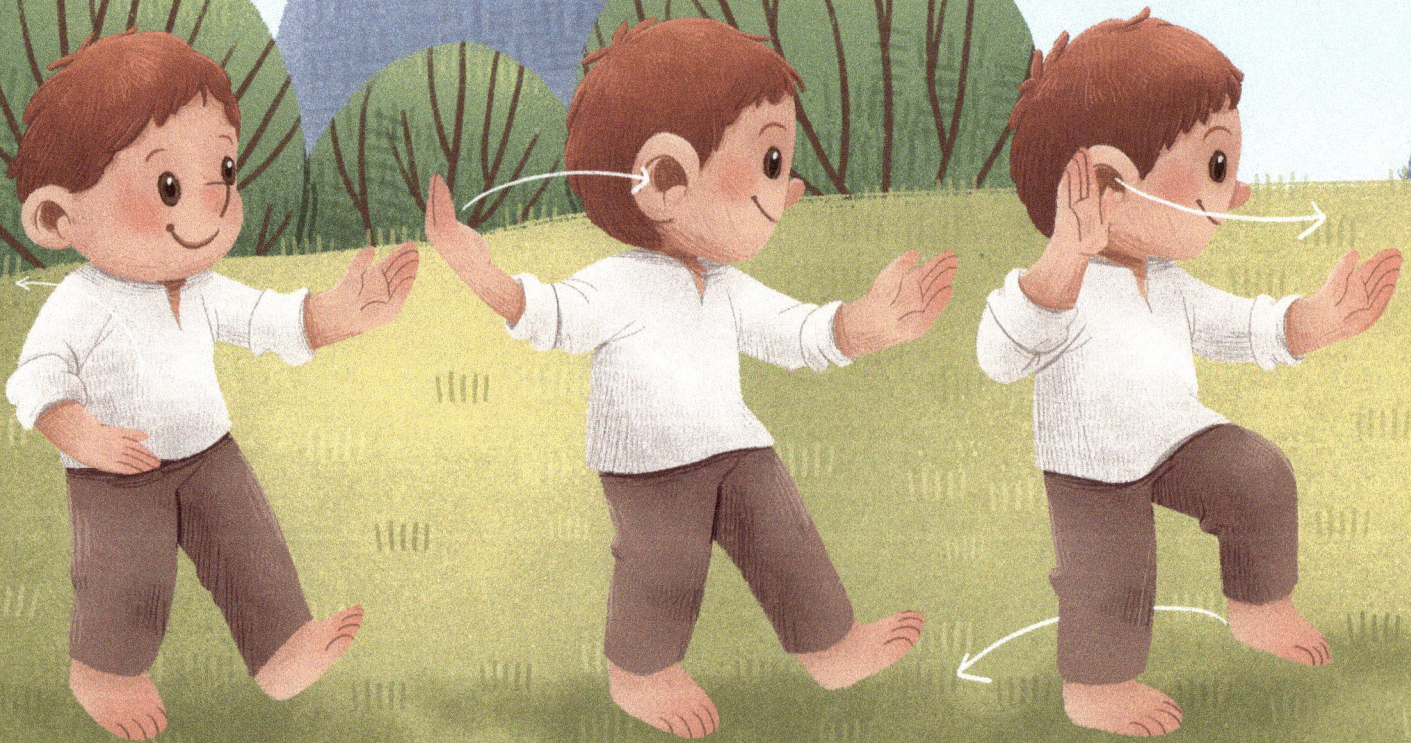

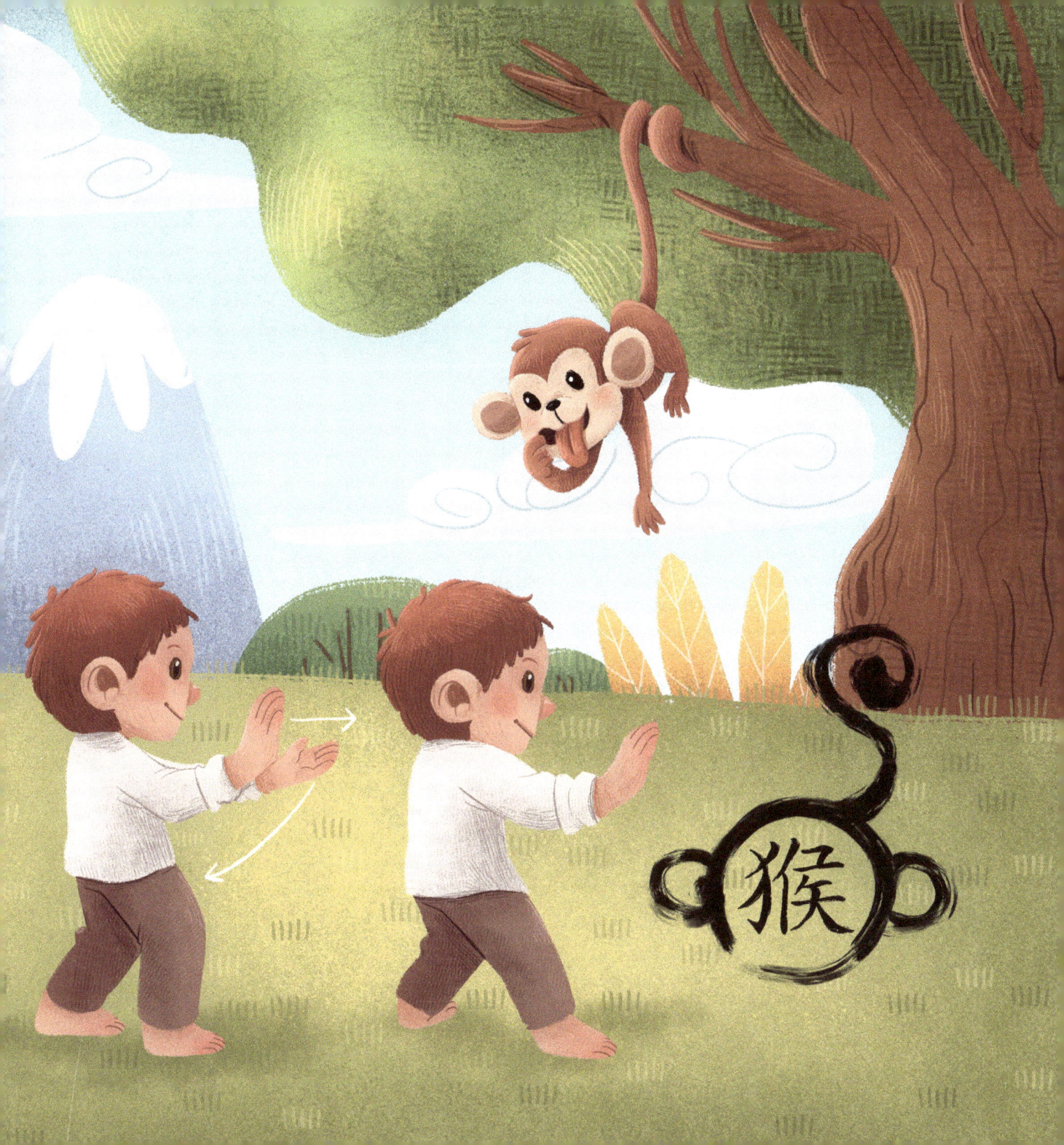

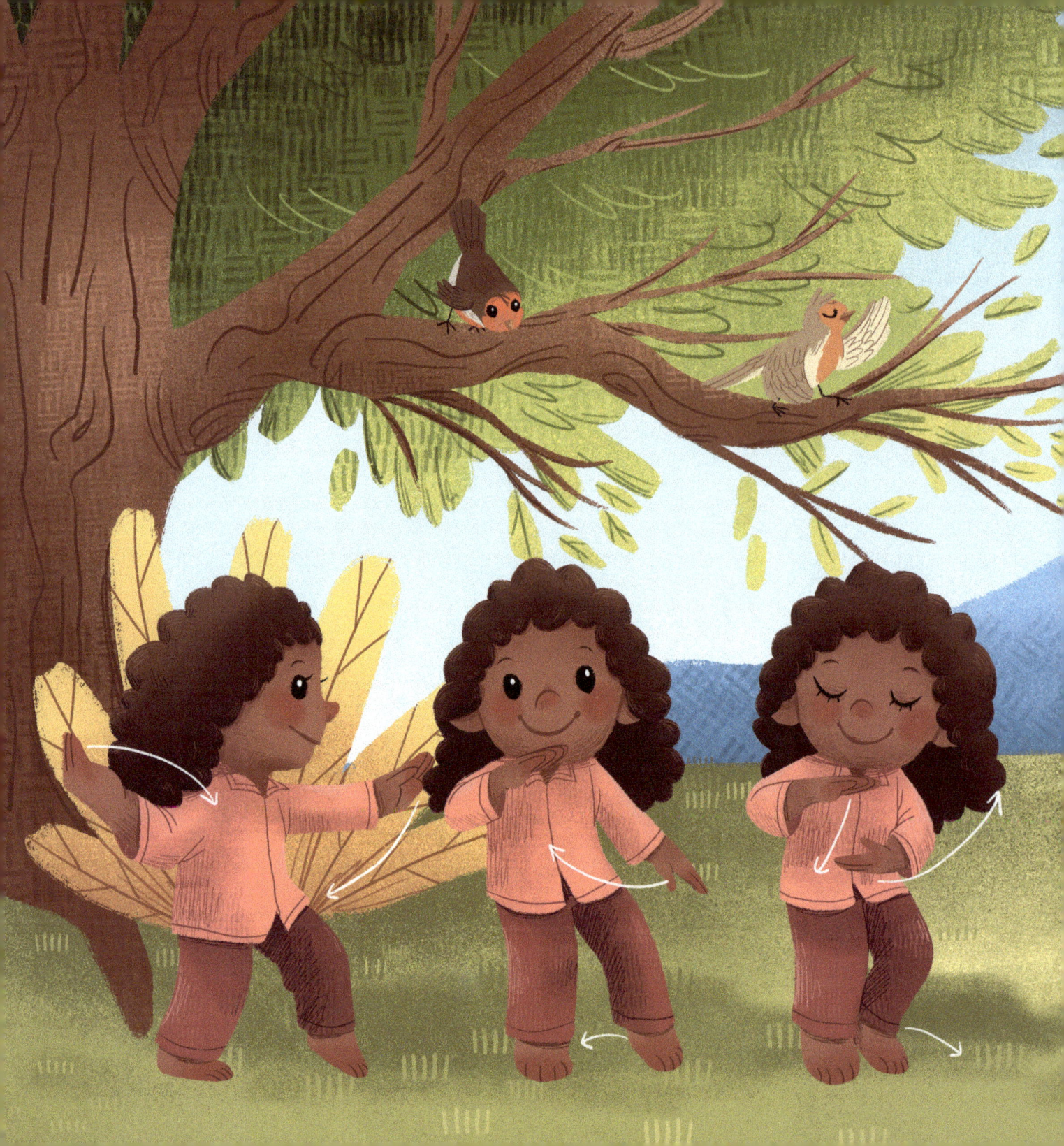

Good morning, little **bird**,
so bright and cheery!

My arms out, reaching
towards your joyful chirping.

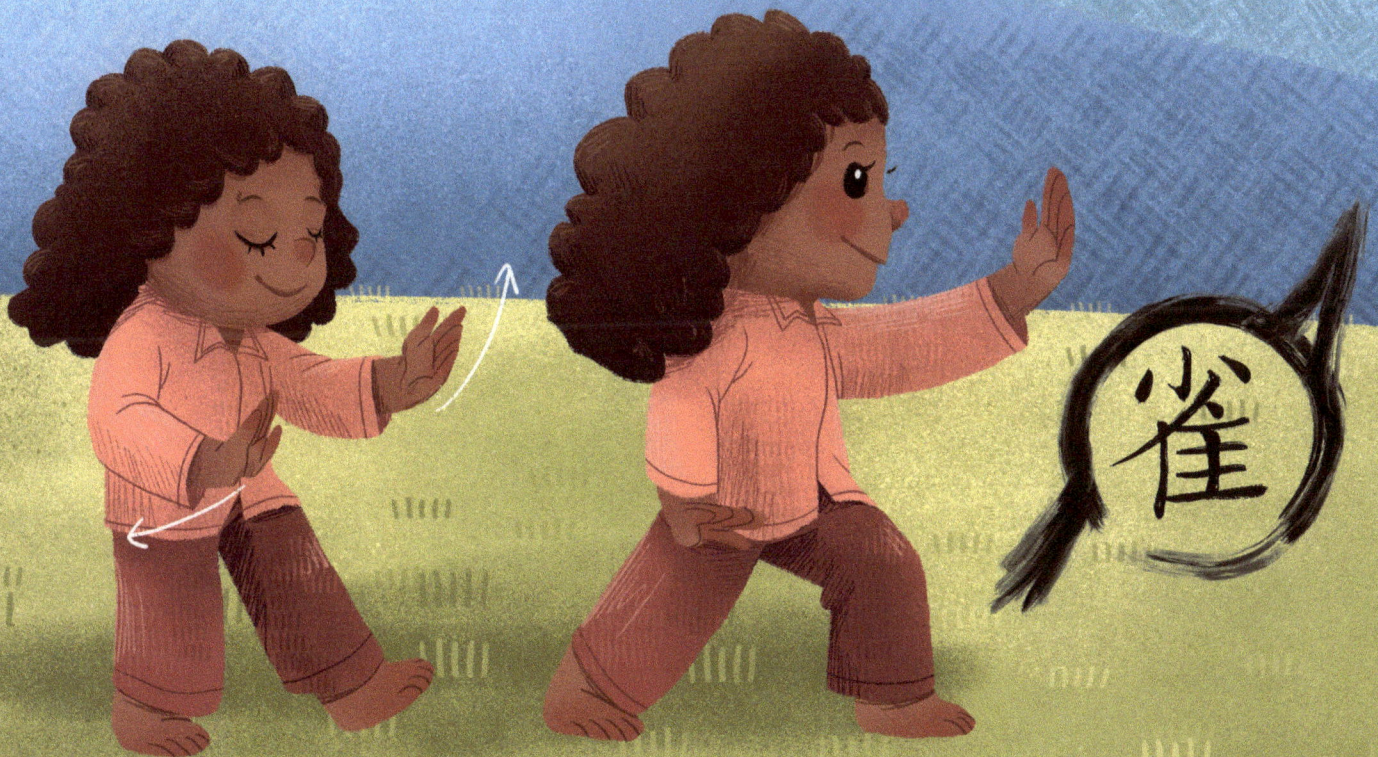

雀

White fluffy clouds, above my head, below my feet, floating all around me!

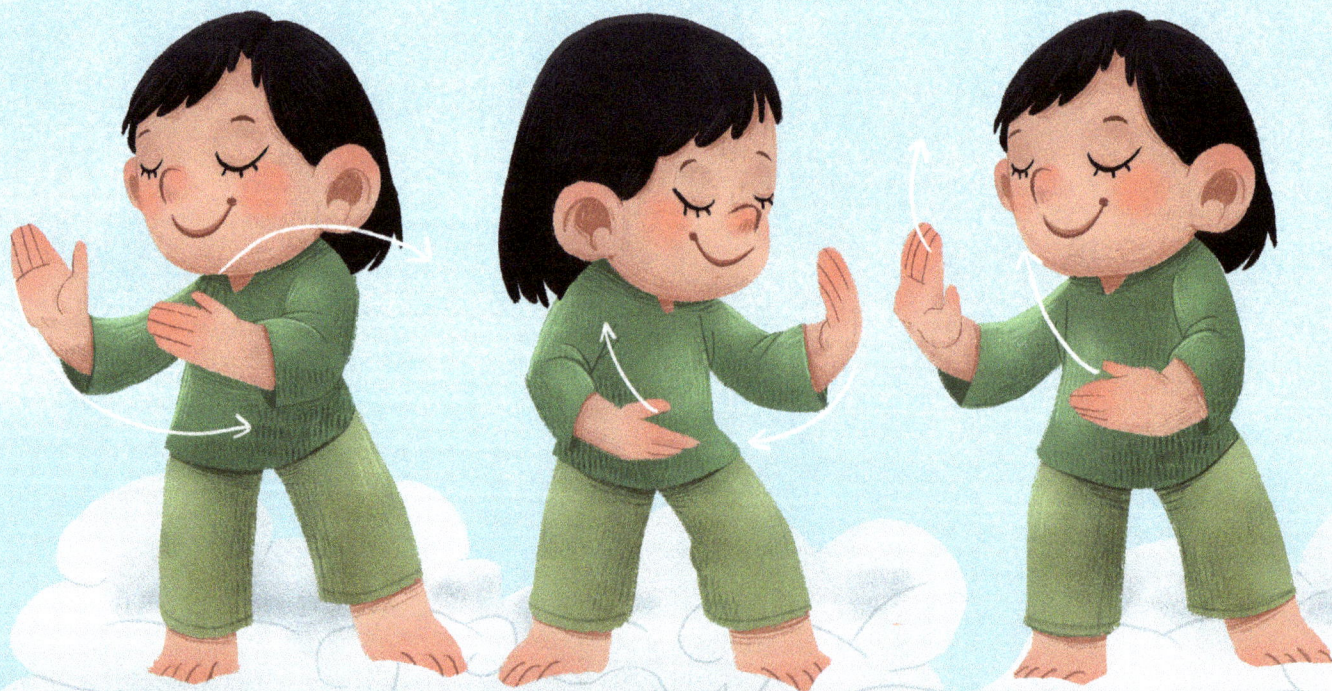

Clouds move me. But, watch,
I can move the clouds, too!

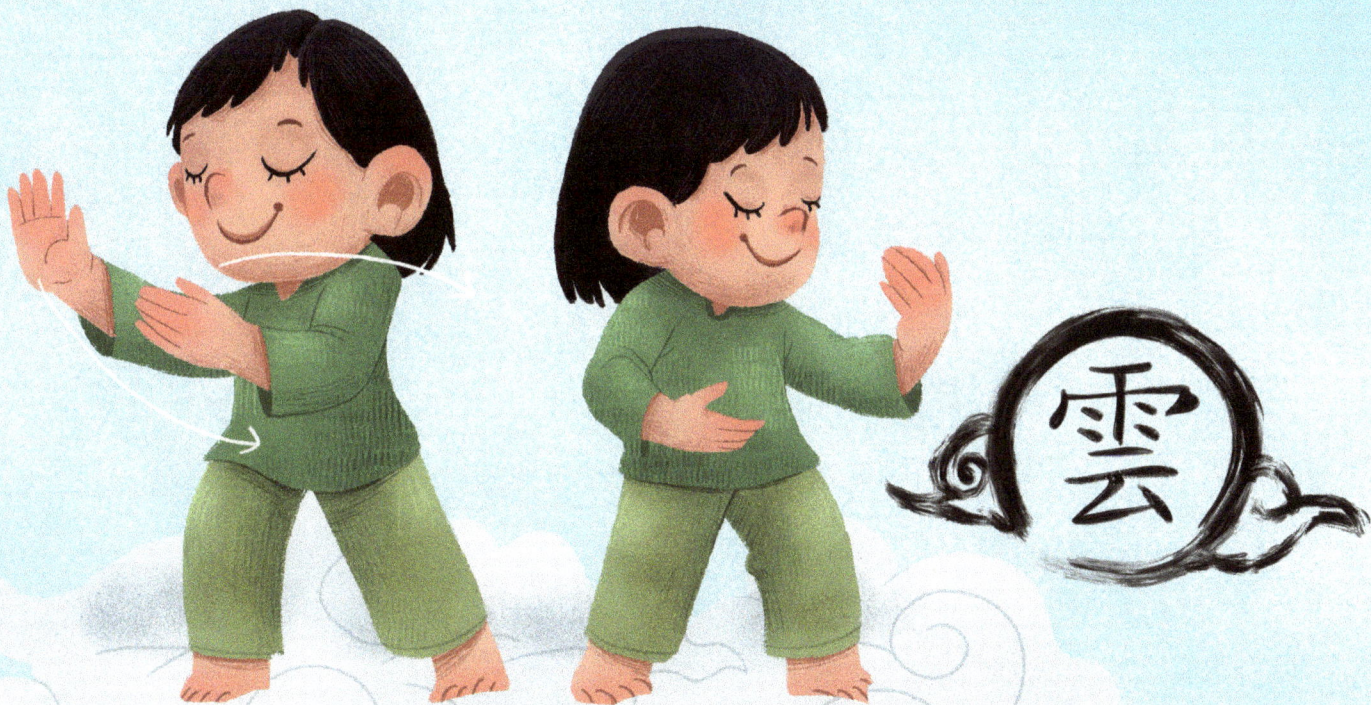

雲

Little **snake**, creeping down,
while I lie low and be still.

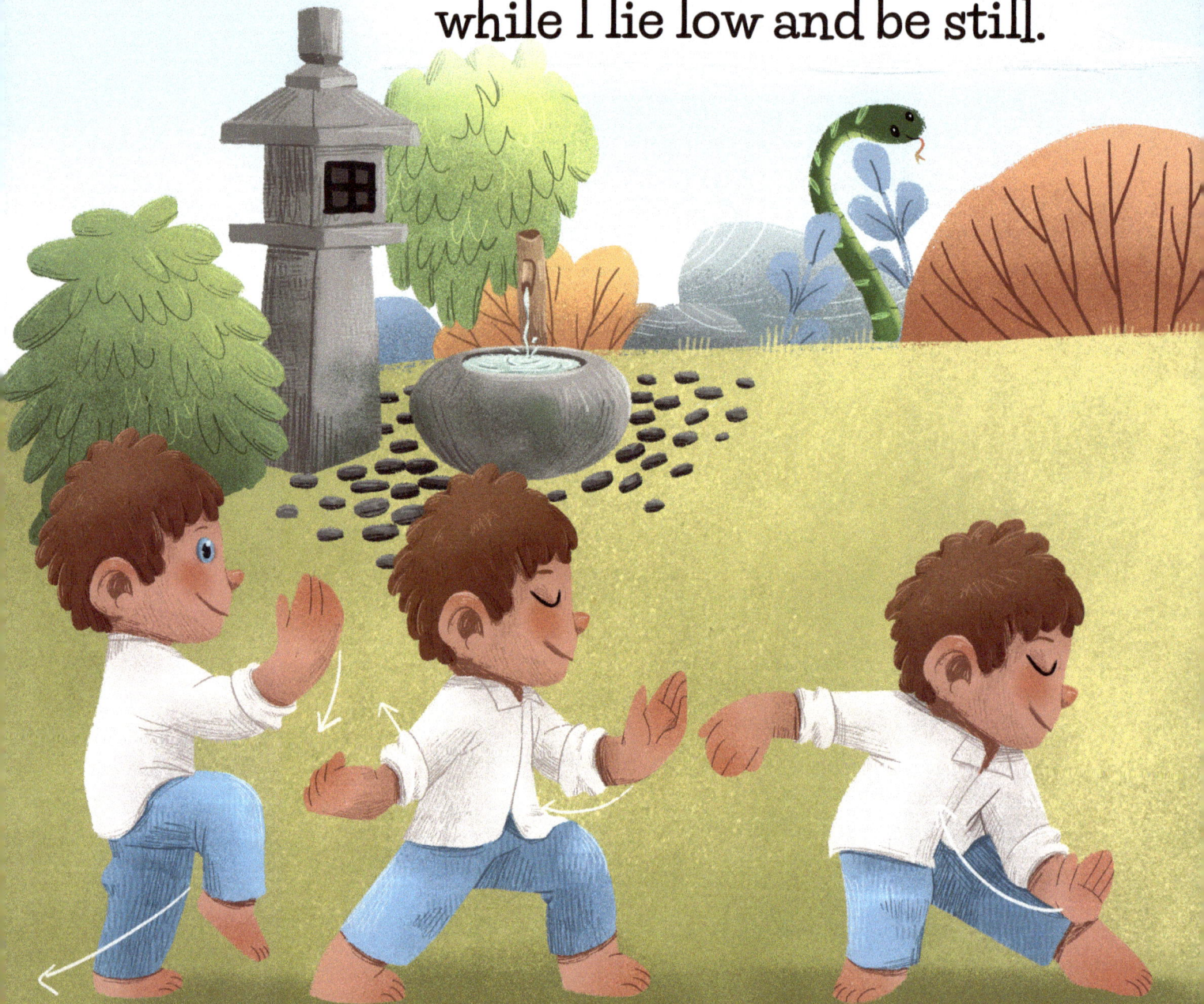

Up and down I move. Left and right I swing. Come and play hide-and-seek with me, little snake. Peekaboo!

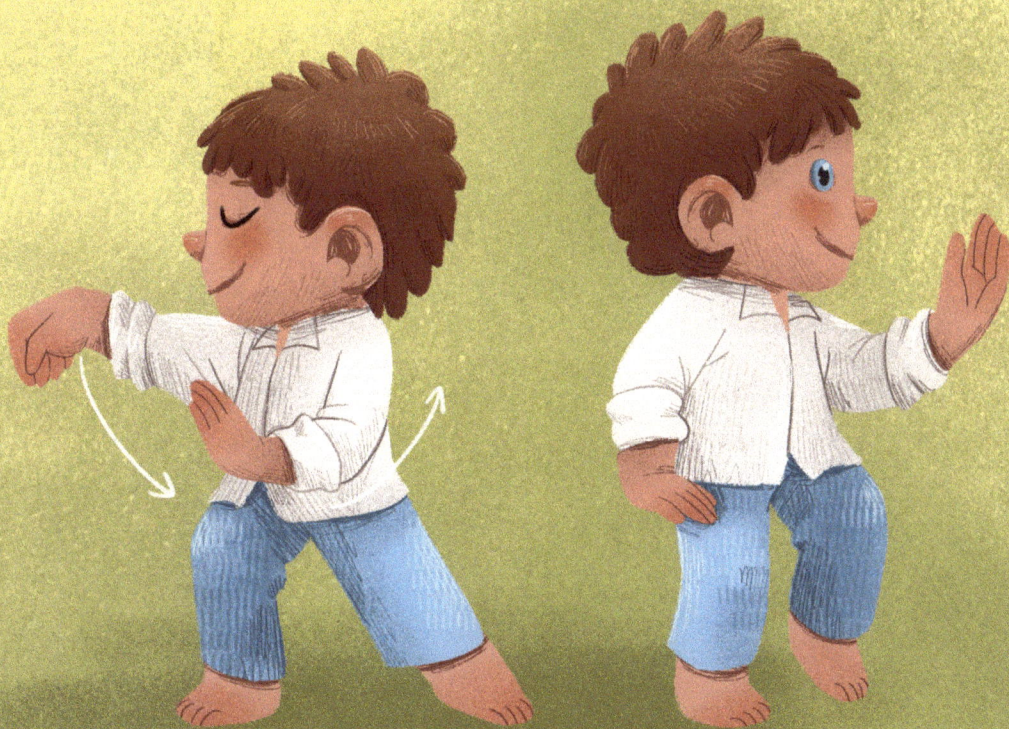

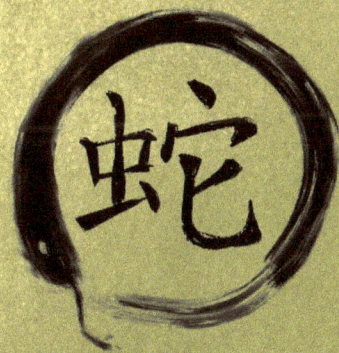

蛇

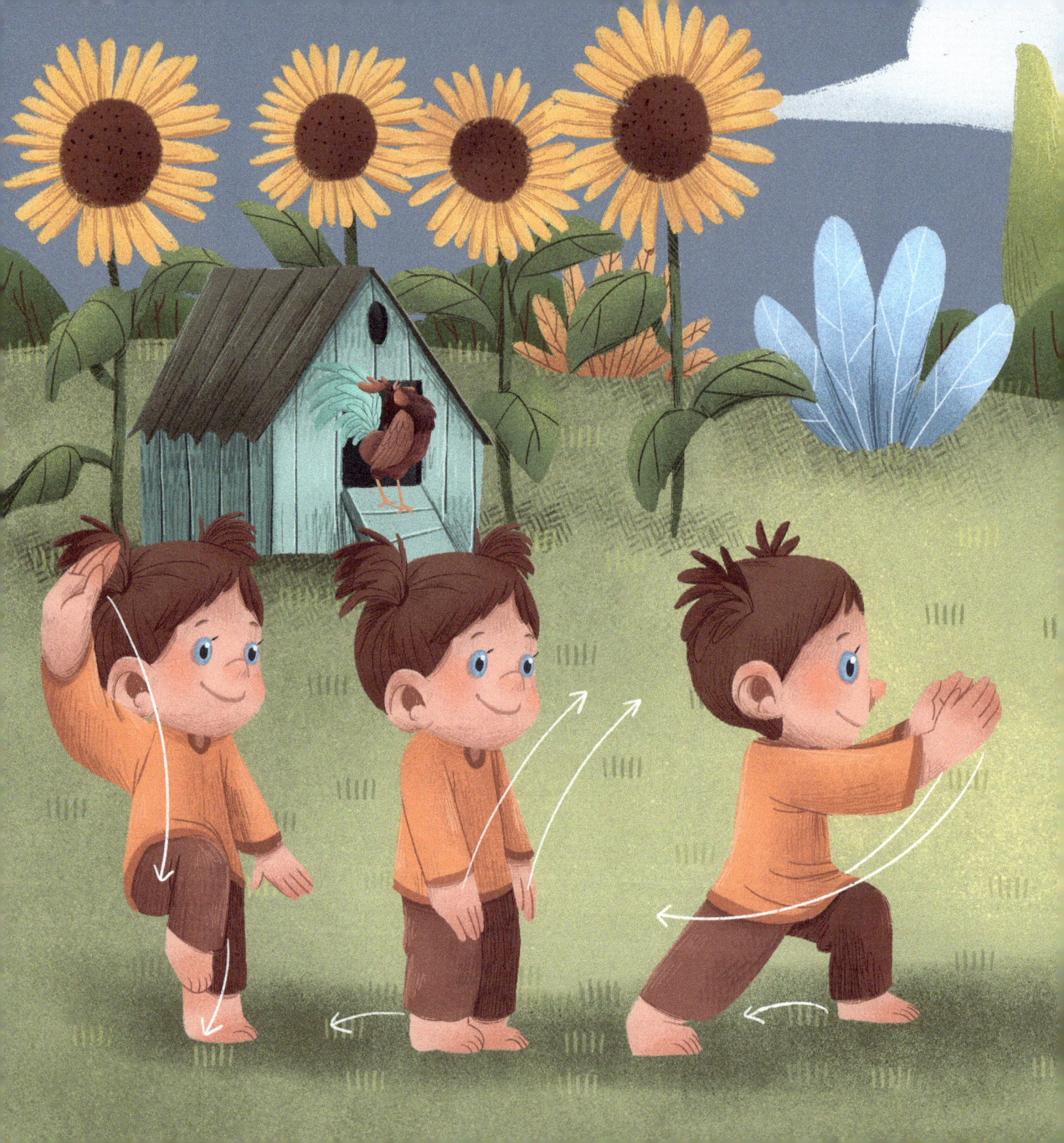

Golden **rooster**, cock-a-doodle-doo!

Good morning, golden sun!
Raise my arm, waving to a
brand new dawn.

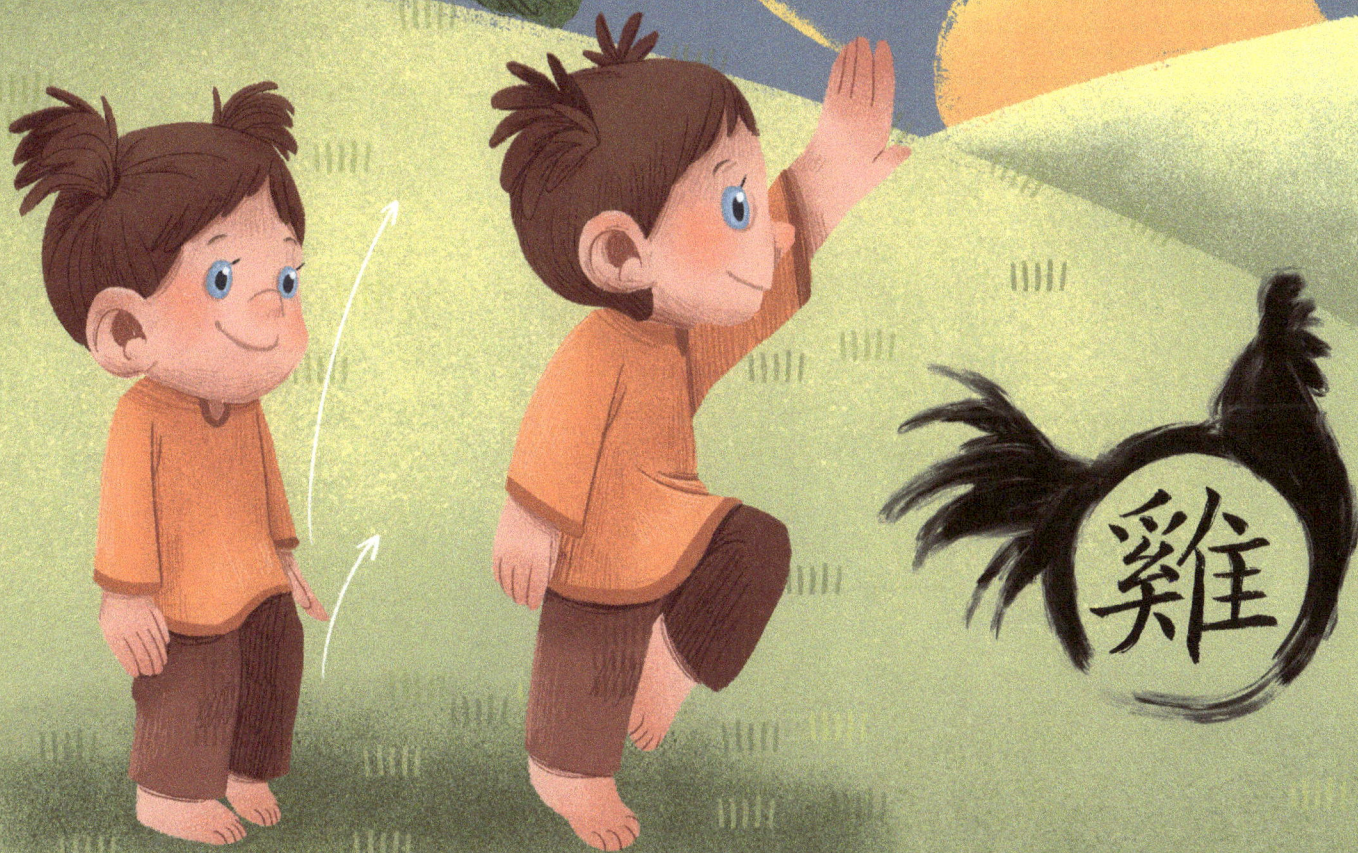

雞

Mighty red **dragon**,
zooms into the clouds,
dives into the ocean,
swirls all around.

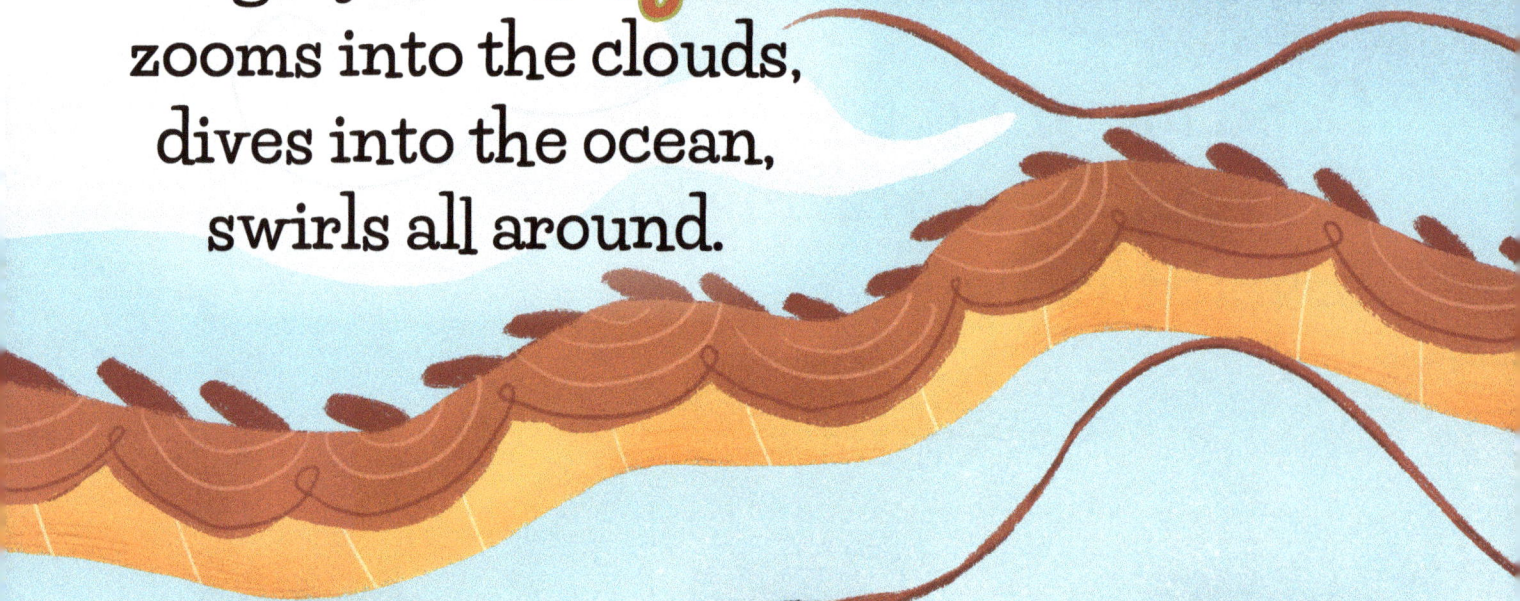

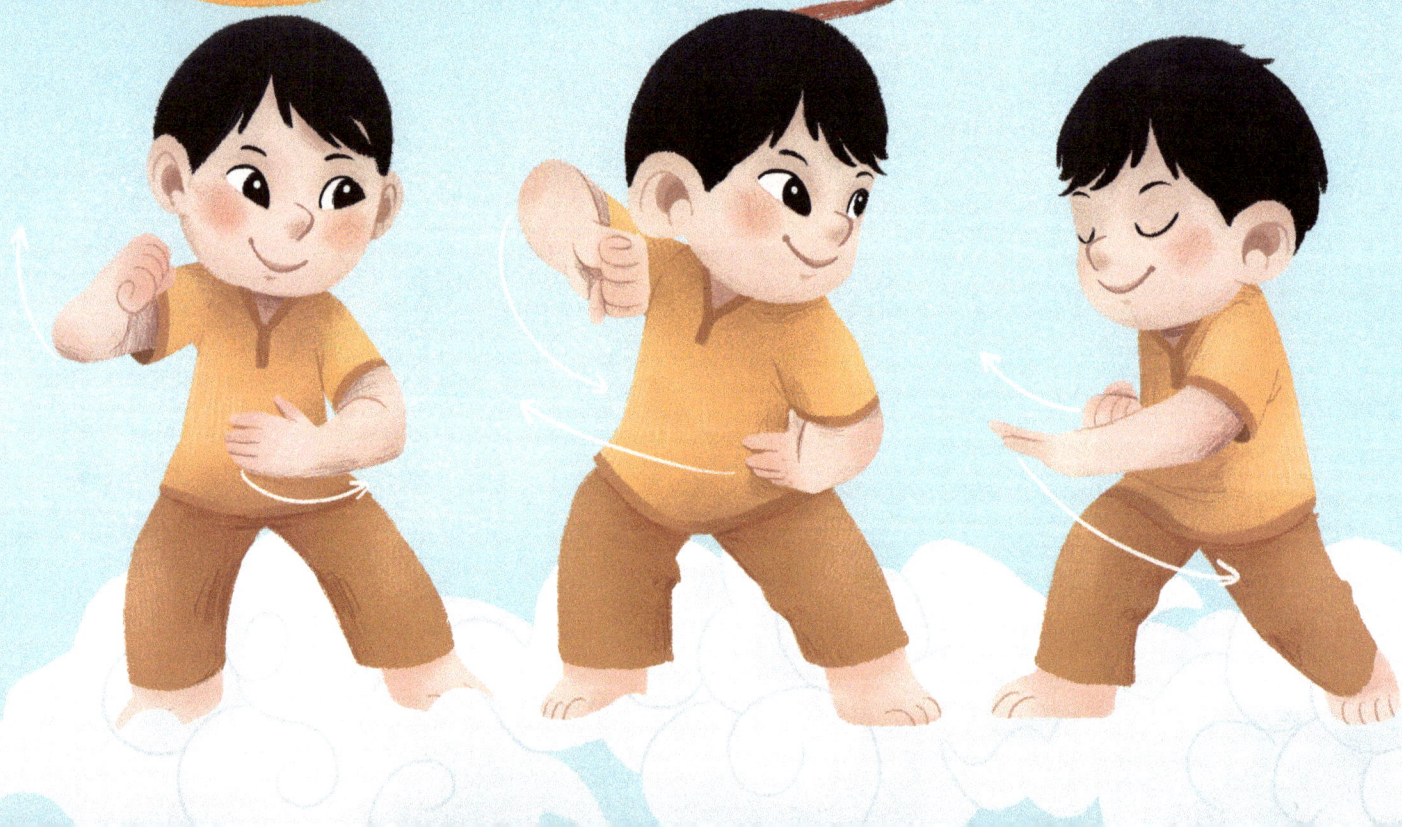

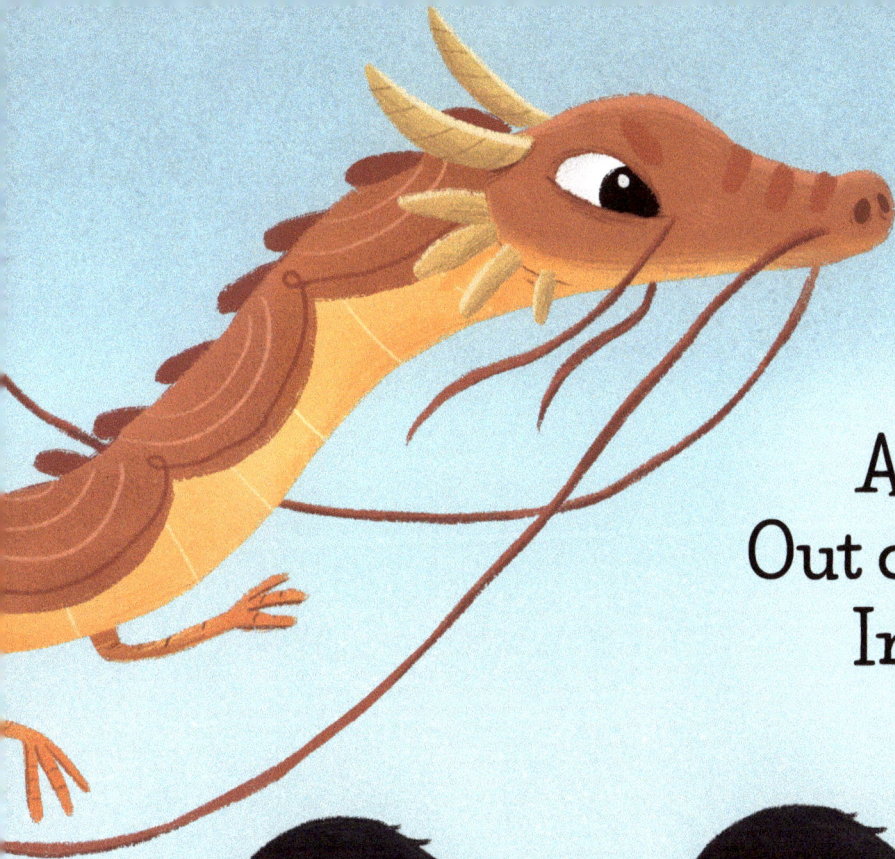

I can follow.
And I can lead.
Out of the sea, I swim.
Into the clouds,
I speed!

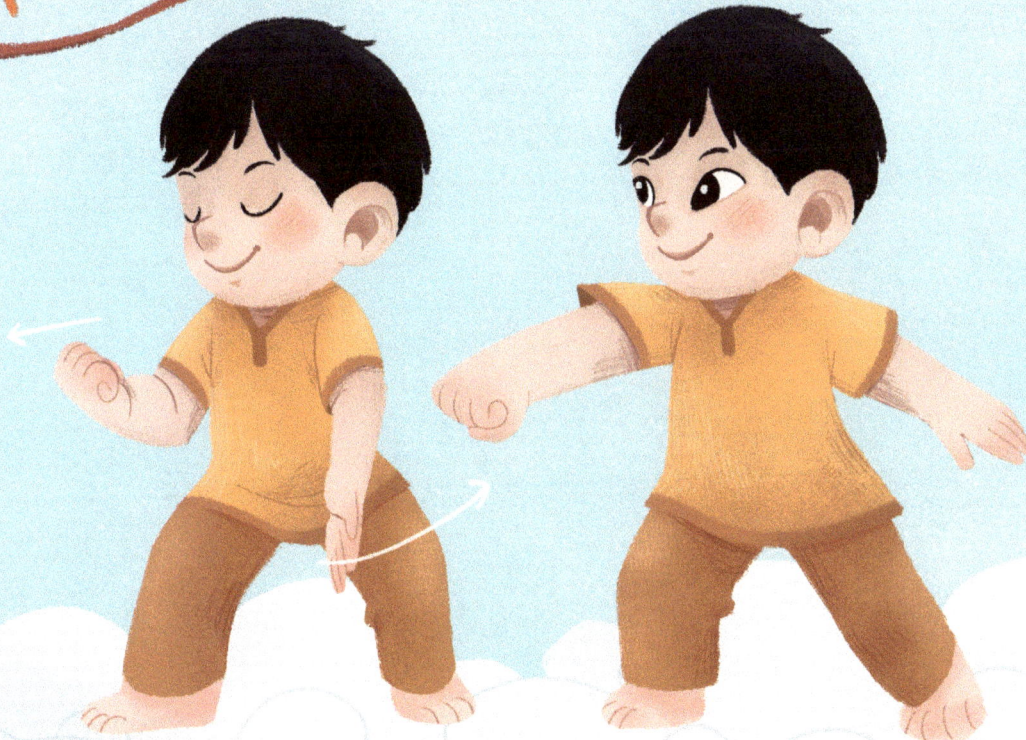

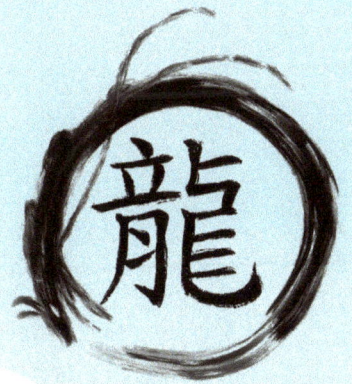

龍

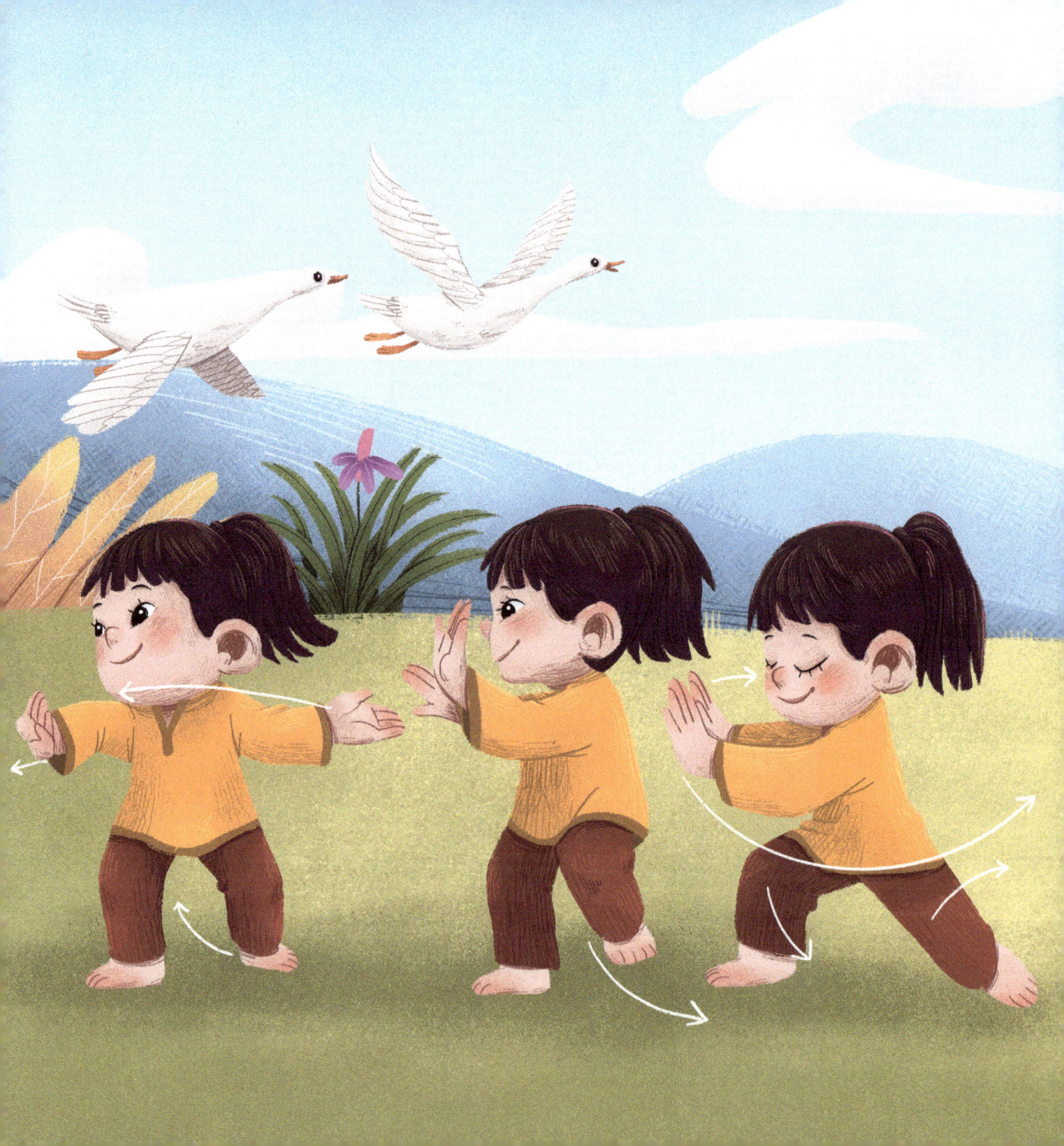

Wild geese flap their wings.
Up, up, up towards the blue sky.

My wings are spread.
I'm ready to fly, too!

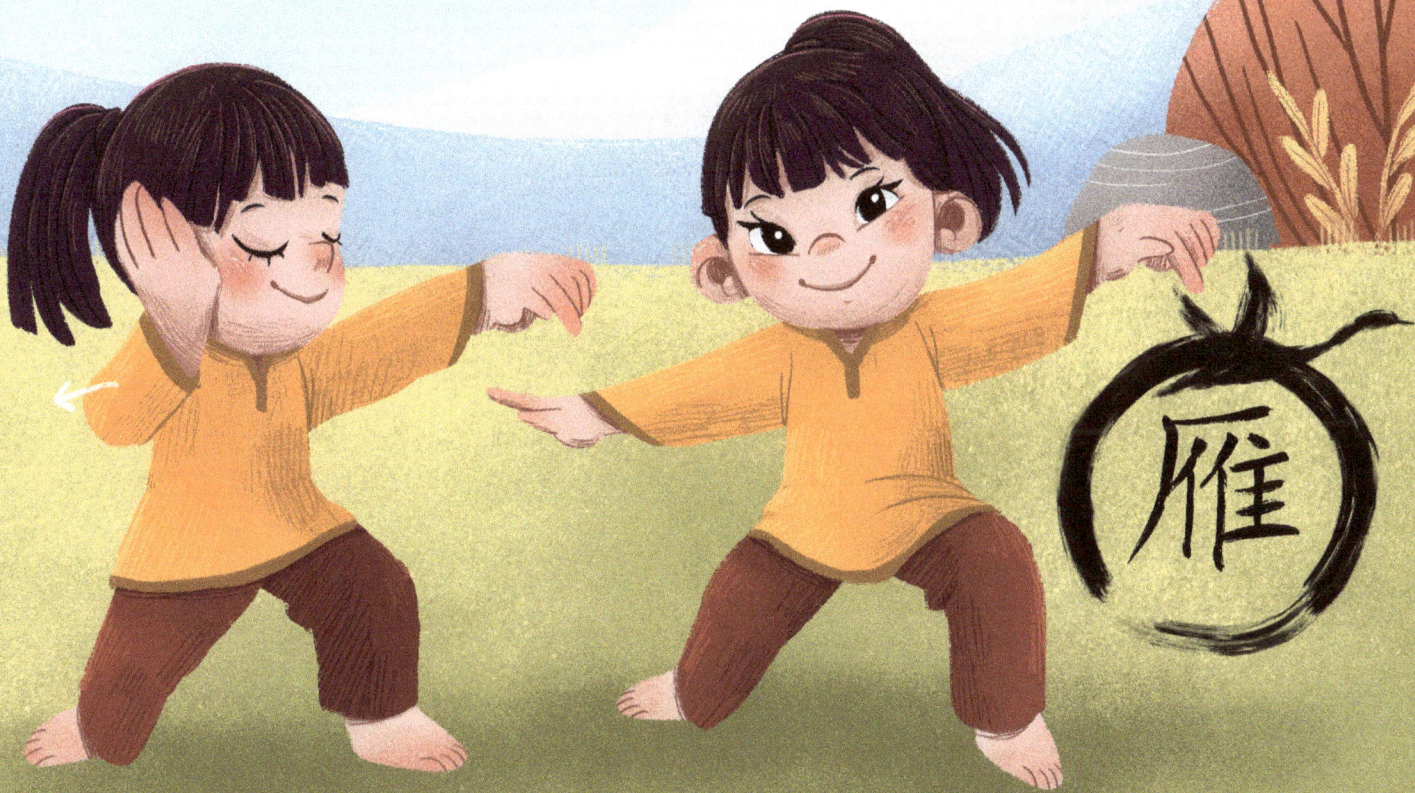

雁

Heavy **tiger**, with legs so big, slowly strolls back to the mountain.

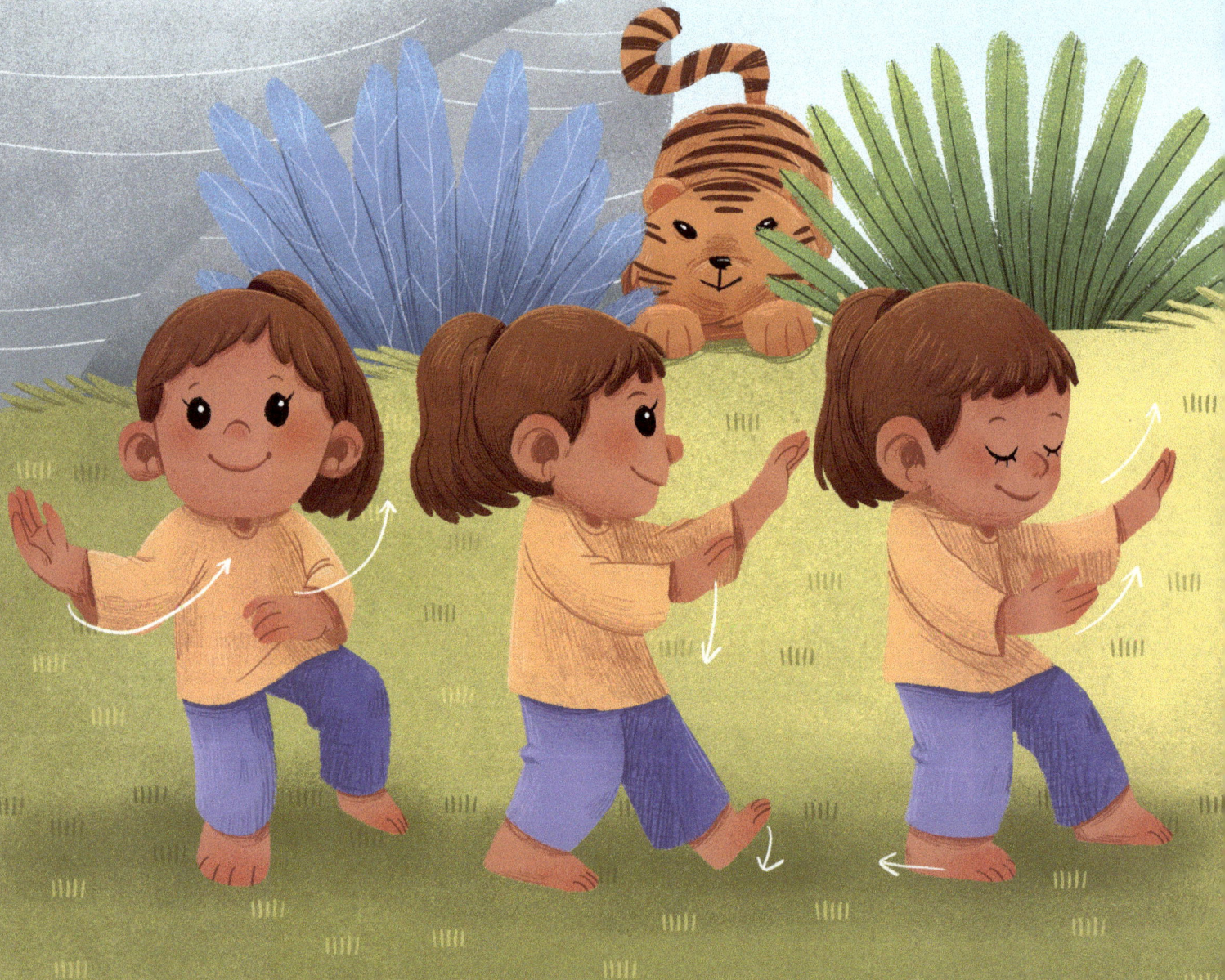

I swing my arms, and stride across the grass.
I embrace the tiger, and return
to the mountain, too.

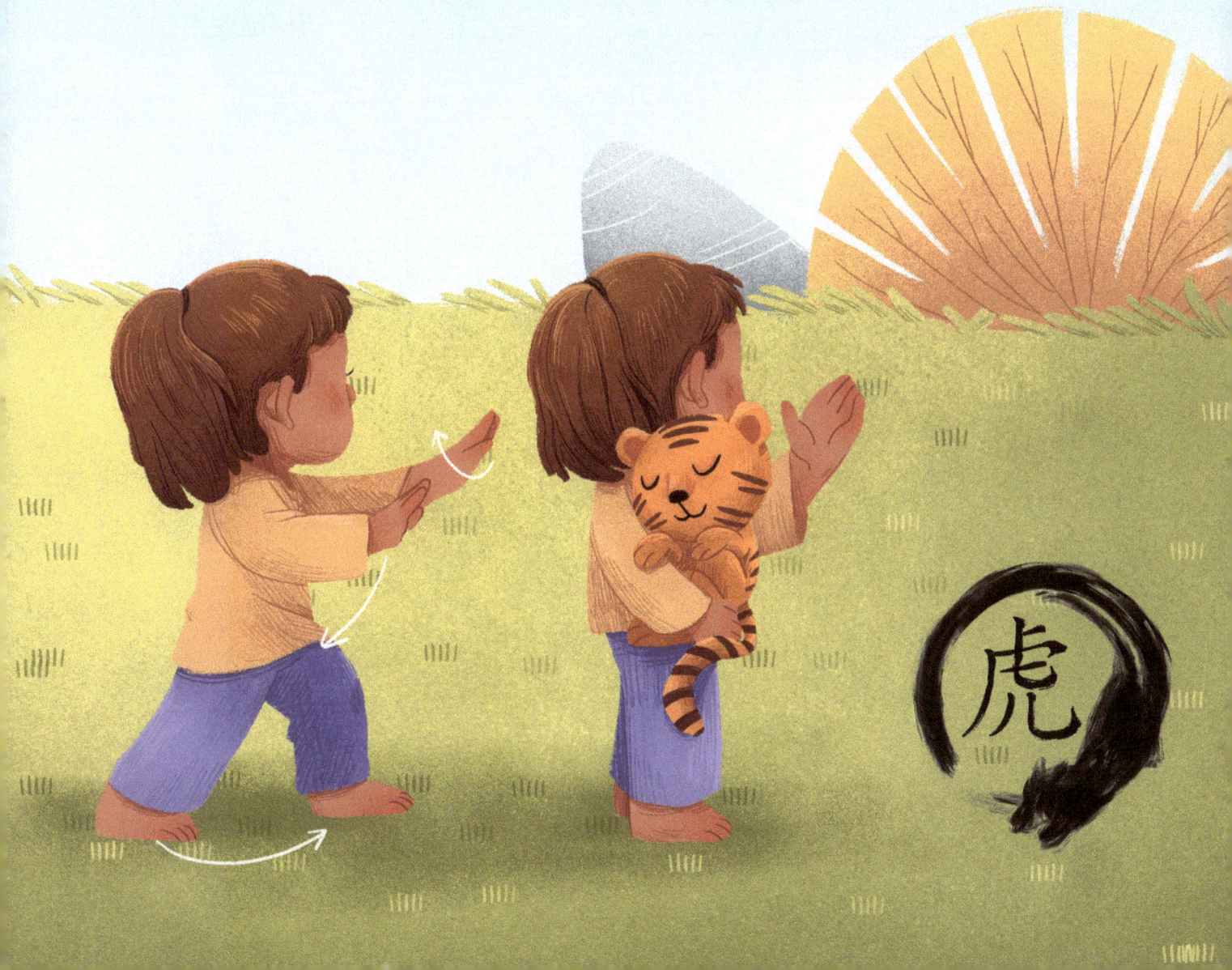

Praying mantis
on a moon-lit night.
Ready, set, go!

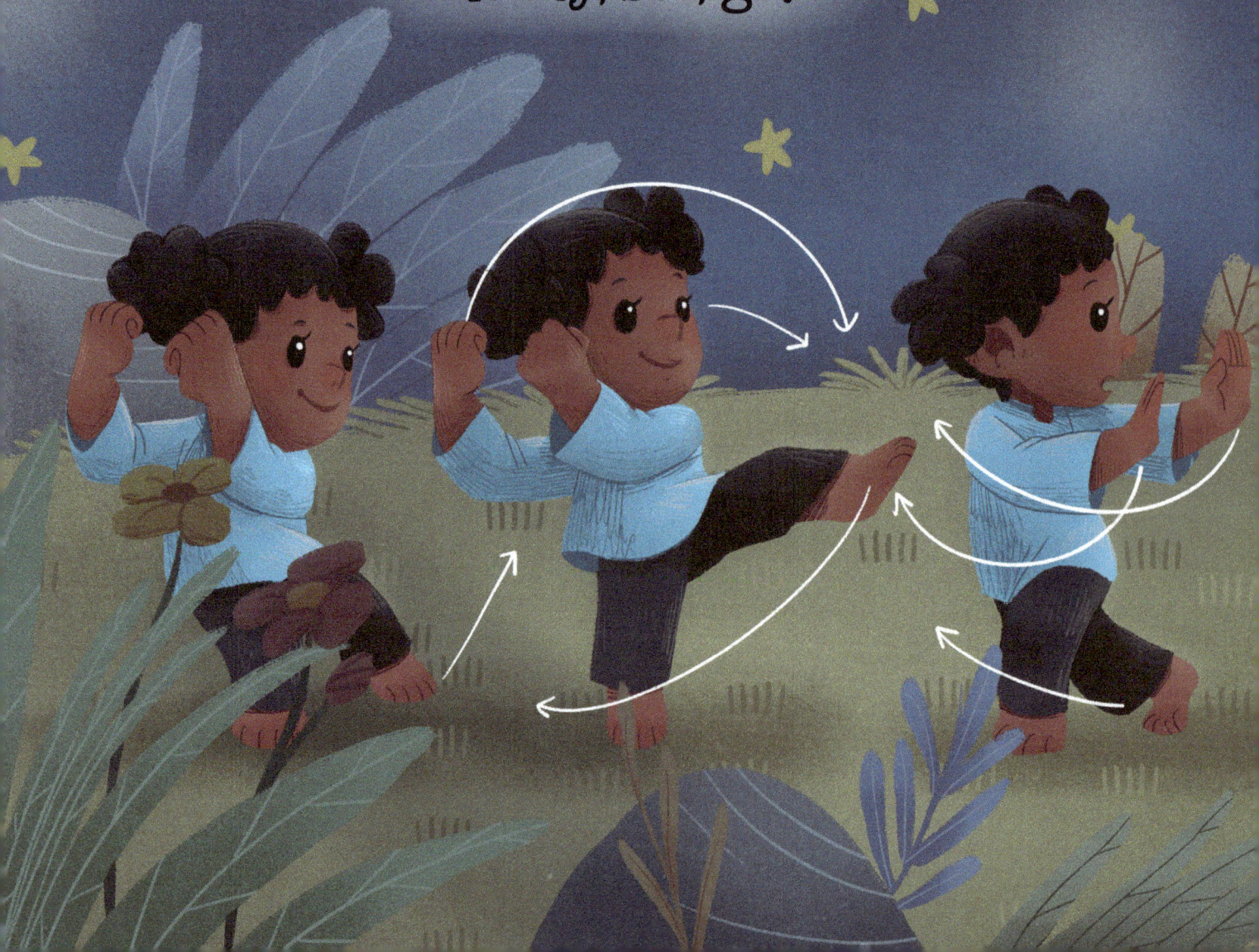

With grace and precision, I am ready to leap forward, too!

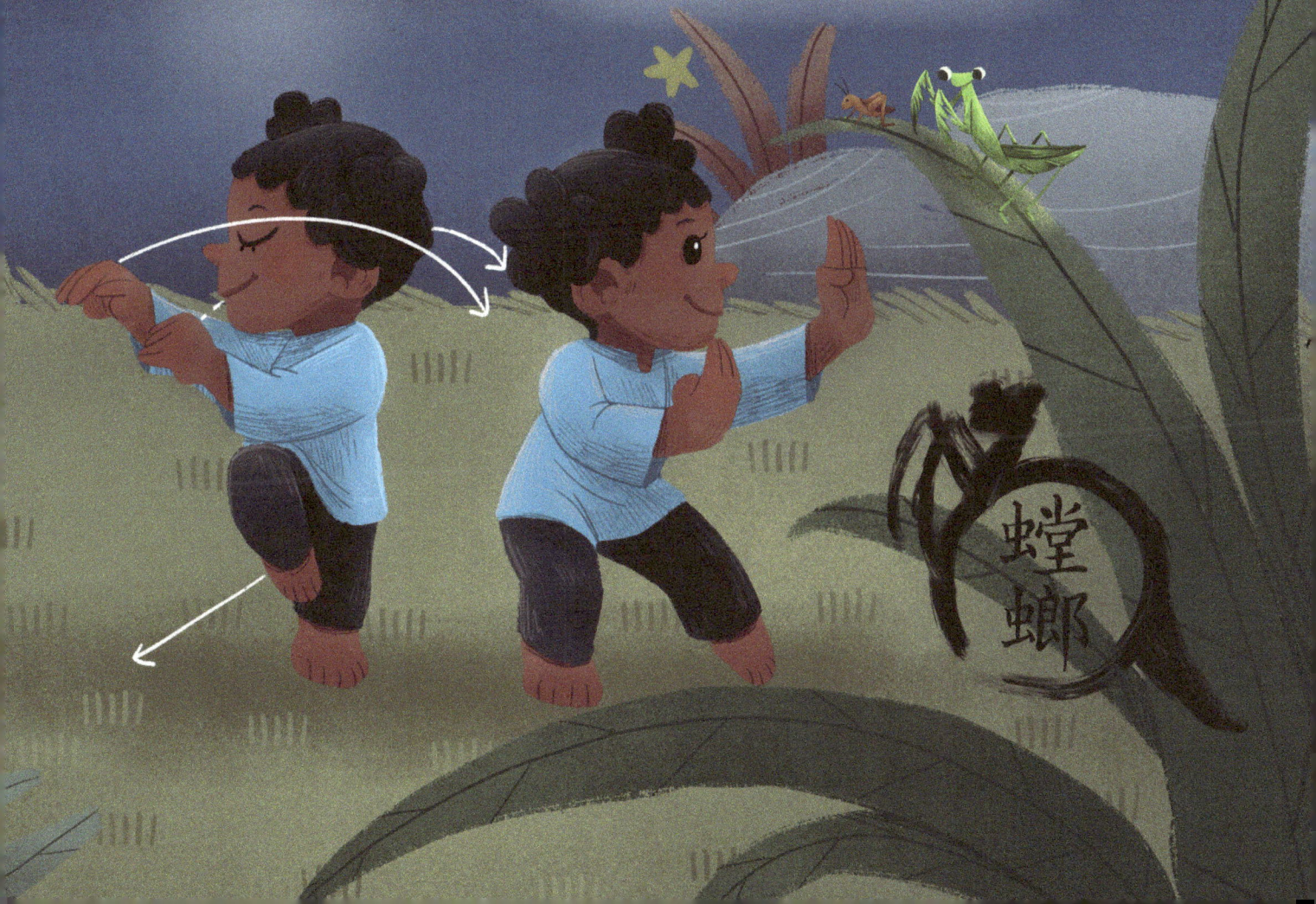

螳螂

Slowly, I take a nice and deep breath in and out, helping the little **dandelion** seeds fly to faraway places.

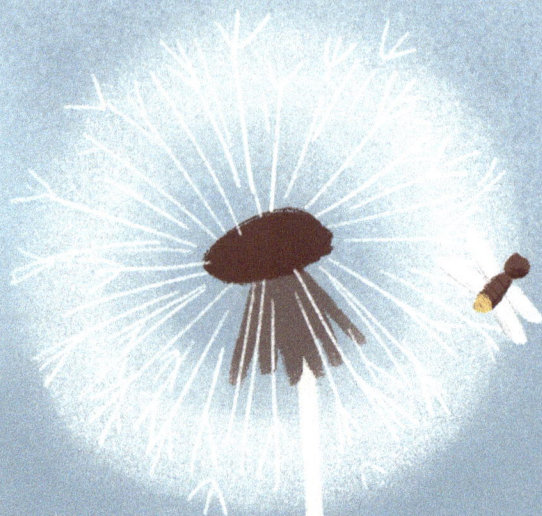

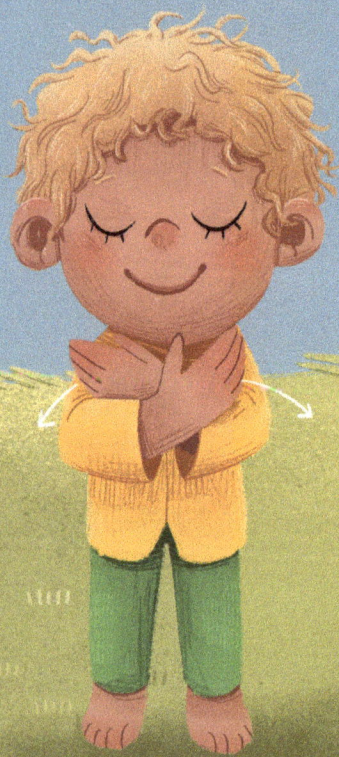

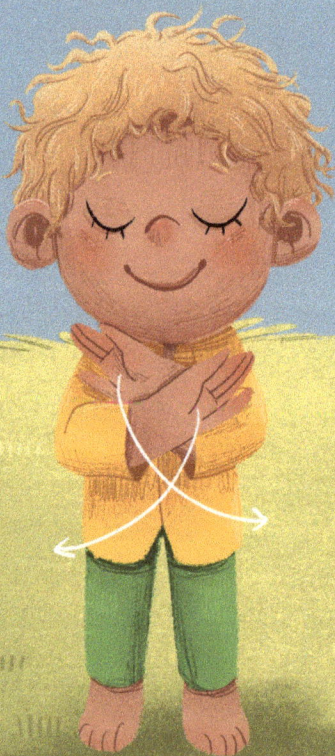

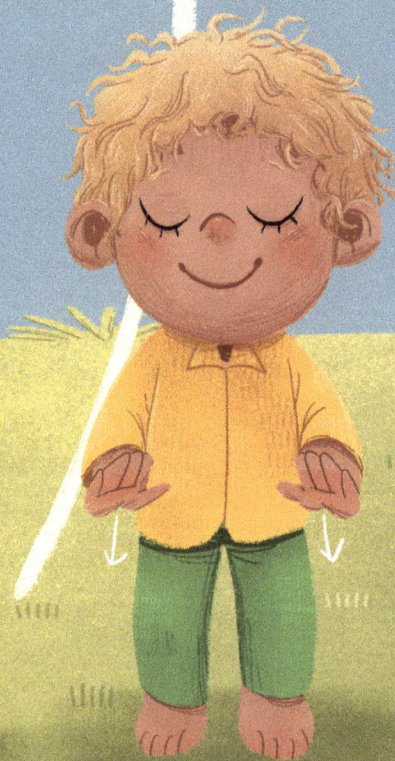

Time to give myself a big hug. Thank you, my strong arms, strong legs, and strong body!

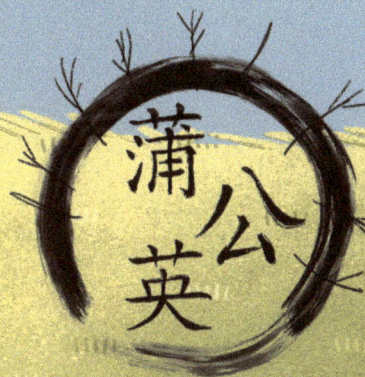

蒲公英

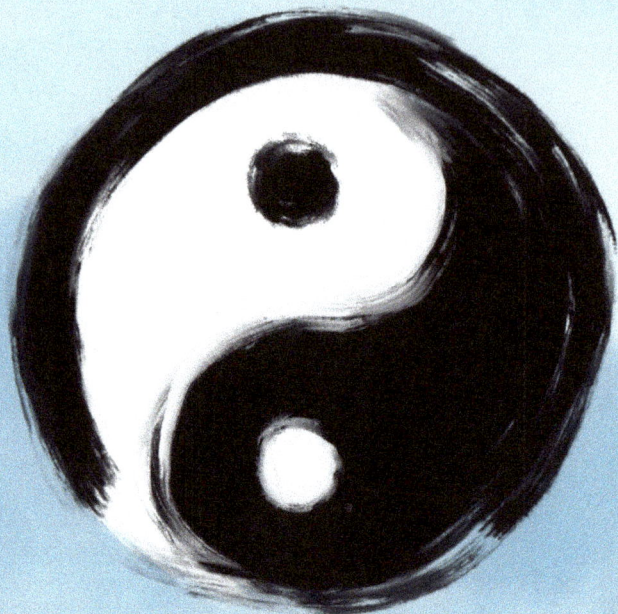

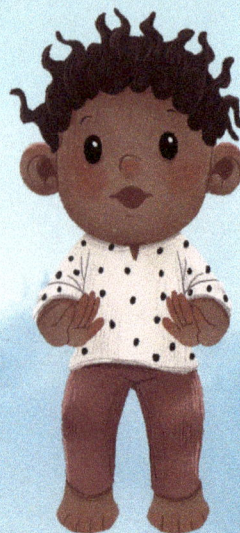

Opening Exercise

Feet, shoulder-width apart, rooting deeply into the earth.

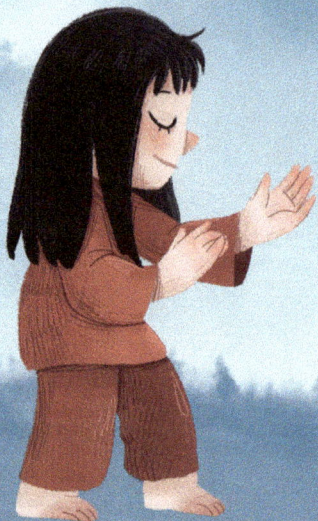

Play the Lute

Arms up, ready to play a sweet melody.

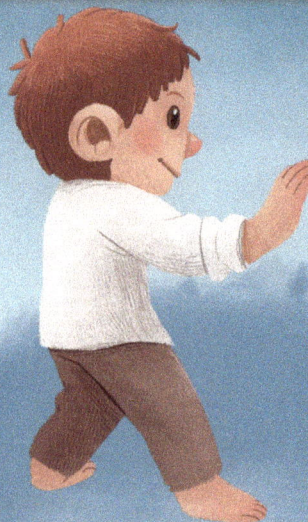

Repulse Monkey

Arms and legs forward. Watch out for the little monkey!

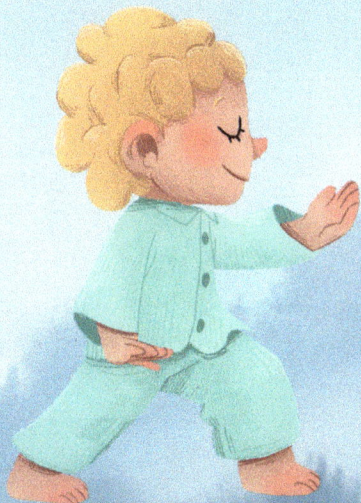

Wild Horse Parts Mane

Arms out and reaching for
the sprinting horse. There it is!

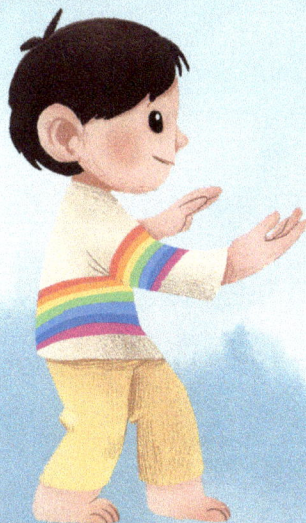

White Crane Spreads its Wings

Legs bent and wings spread,
flying like a crane!

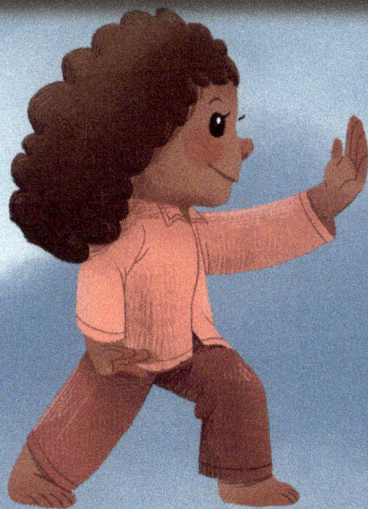

Bird's Tail

Legs bent, reaching out to
the cheerful little bird.

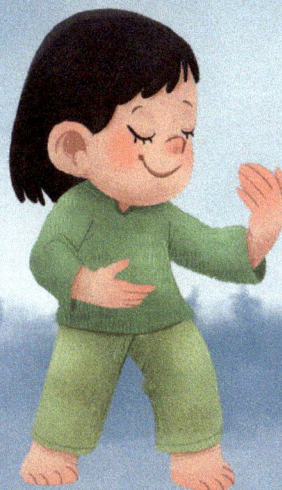

Hands in the Cloud

Hands in the cloud,
moving in a circulation motion.

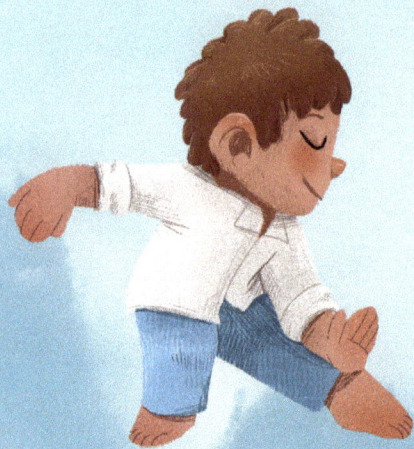

Snake Creeps Down

Bent down low,
and arms like a little snake. Hiss!

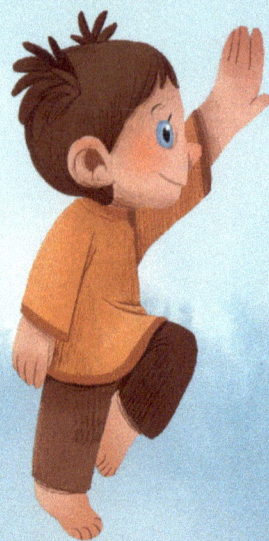

Golden Rooster Stands on One Leg

Leg up, and waking up early,
with the rooster who crows at sunrise.

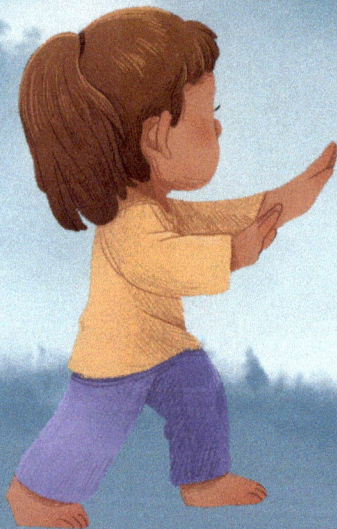

Embrace Tiger, Return to Mountain

Legs bent, ready to pounce, grrr!

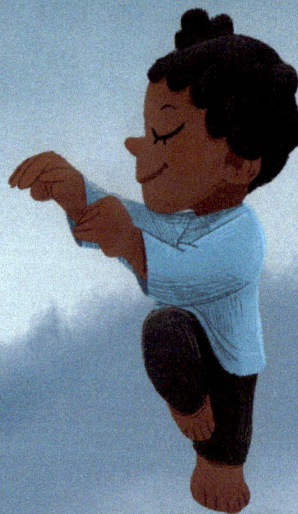

Praying Mantis on the Move

Hands together, leg up and down,
leaping like a praying mantis!

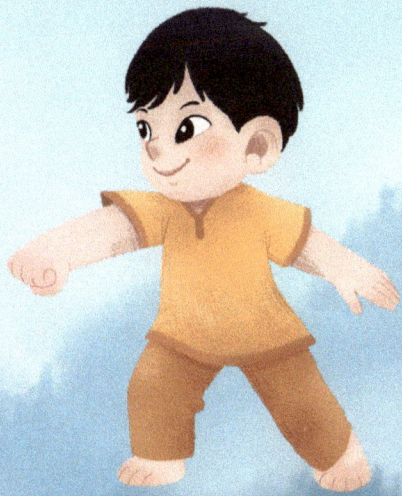

Dragon Flies out of Water

Fist clenched and arms spread,
flying like a dragon.

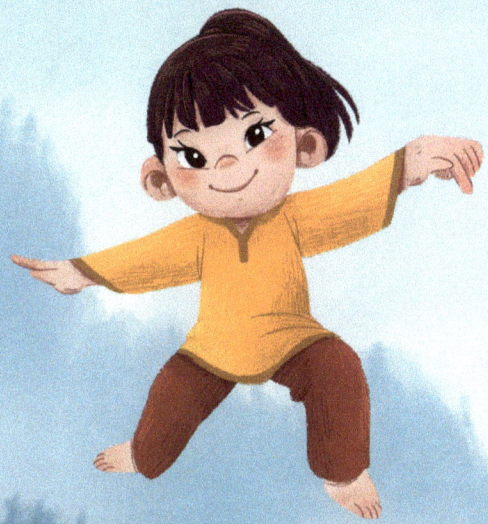

Wild Goose Flies Away

Legs out, shoulder-width.
Arms up and flap your wings!

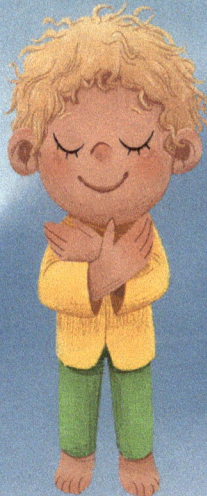

Closing Exercise

Hug yourself and give thanks to your
strong body. Breathe in and out slowly.

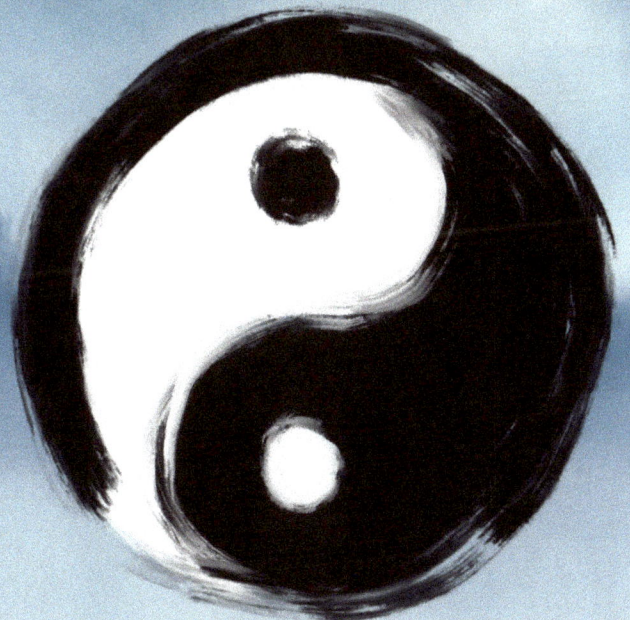

Words for Parents and Caregivers

Greetings, parents and caregivers! You're about to embark on an exciting journey as you and your children learn about the ancient Chinese art of tai chi. This martial art is practiced for its life energy and health benefits by millions of people worldwide, both young and old. Research studies show that tai chi can help reduce stress, heart disease, high blood pressure, and many other ailments.

The creator of tai chi was a Daoist monk, who knew that moving the body in special ways would bring inner peace and tranquility. Think of tai chi as a form of "*meditation in motion*". Practicing tai chi allows you to experience *stillness in motion* and to build a more harmonic mind-body connection. Modern lifestyle often results in too much movement in the mind and too much stillness in the body, causing an unbalanced internal state of Yin and Yang energy. By directing your awareness inward and focusing on your breathing and bodily sensations, you can tune into the flow of energy from within and stay in the present moment. Tai chi practice helps still your mind, while it moves your body in a slow, flowing motion.

Many of the tai chi moves are modeled after animals. What better way to introduce children to tai chi, than with the inviting images of cranes, tigers, and even mythical, colorful dragons? This exciting way of introducing healthy body movements and mindful breathing techniques can help build a positive habit that will last a lifetime.

You and your children will soon discover the powerful benefits of tai chi, as it sends good, positive energy throughout your body. That energy is called *qi*. This life energy helps relax you and, in turn, uplifts your spirits.

When you take the time each day to practice, you will start to feel more energized, more mindful, and more balanced. Your mind and body will be healthier. Each move is special in its own way, helping *qi* flow to different parts of the body. You and your family will soon discover why so many people practice tai chi as a way of life.

The Ancient Art is Yours to Practice

Now you, too, parents and children alike, know the incredible benefits of tai chi. You can move like an animal, so gracefully. You are increasing your flexibility, improving your balance, building your strength, boosting your heart health, lowering stress, and enhancing your focus.

Are you a little crane?
Are you chasing a monkey?
Are you a wild goose?

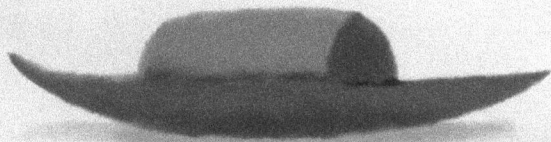

Keep practicing every day, discover your *qi*, and feel all the positive energy flow through you!

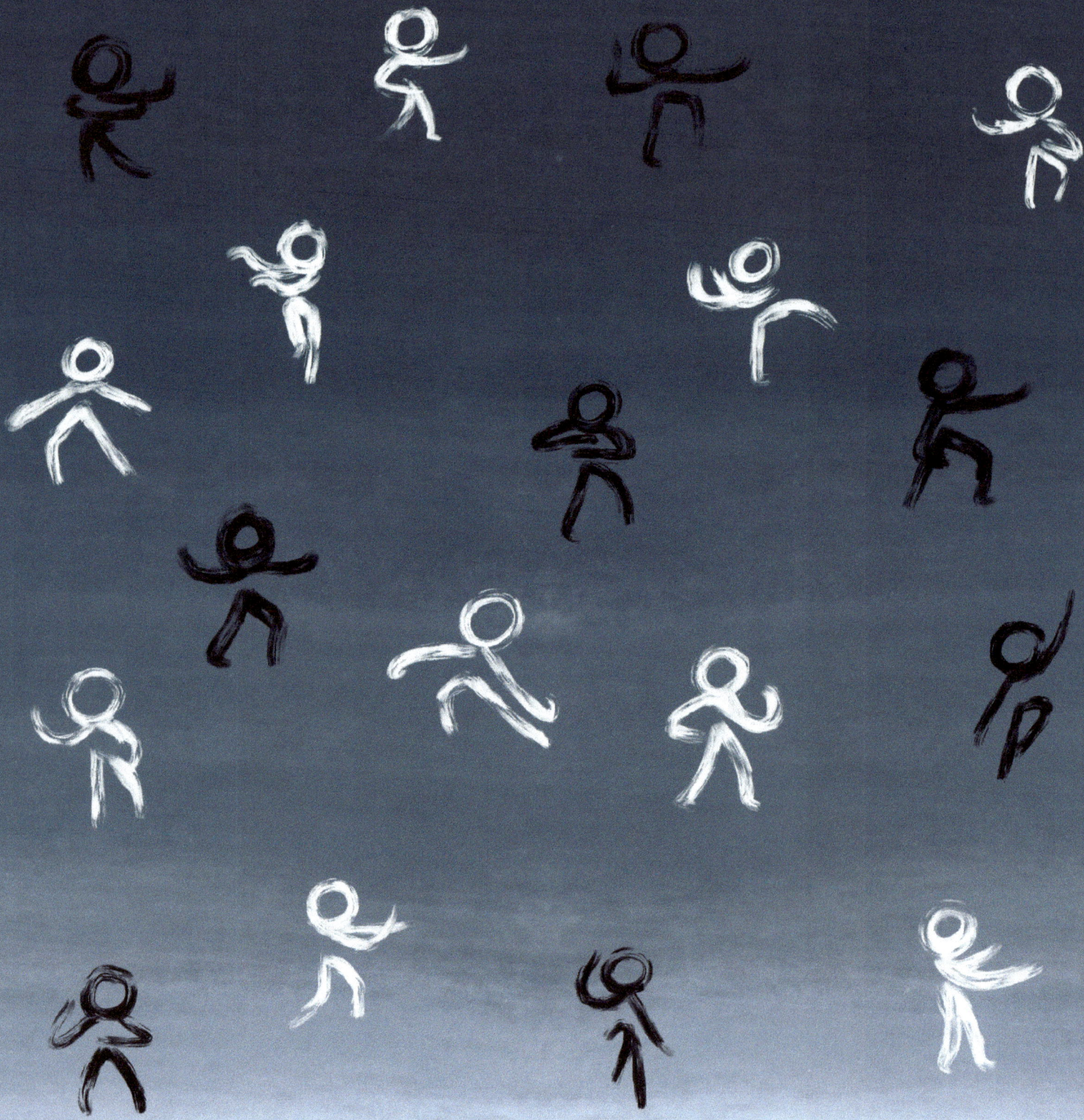

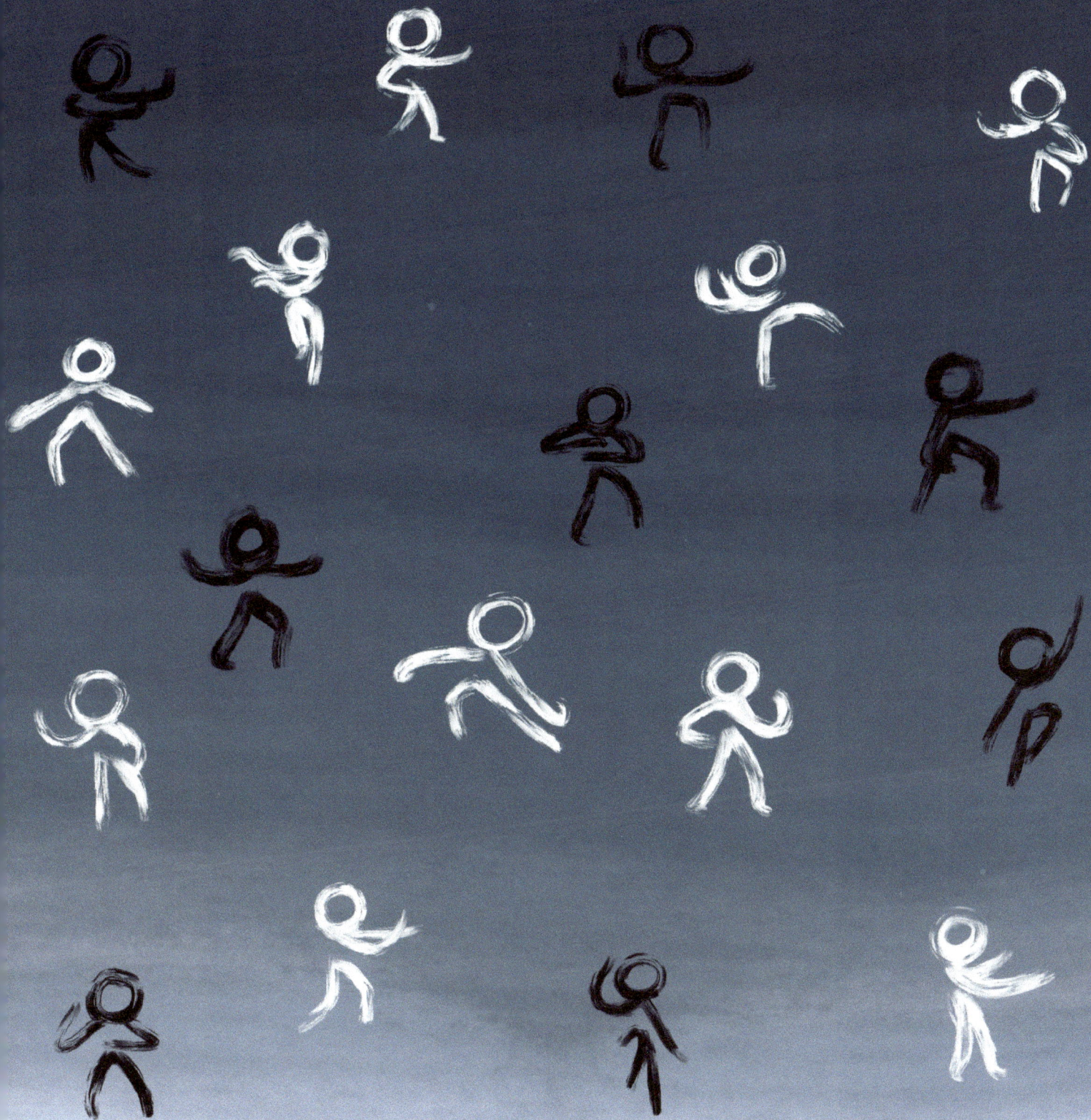

www.ingramcontent.com/pod-product-compliance
Lightning Source LLC
Chambersburg PA
CBHW042355030426

42336CB00029B/3485